Skin Cancer Detection Using Artificial Intelligence Techniques

This book explores the application of artificial intelligence (AI) in diagnosing skin cancer, emphasizing the importance of early detection to improve treatment outcomes. It reviews various Deep Learning (DL) algorithms, with a focus on CNN, to classify skin cancer with higher accuracy than traditional methods. Designed for beginners and experts alike, the book provides a comprehensive understanding of AI techniques and their implementation in healthcare.

- Compares the accuracy of AI-based detection methods with traditional medical practices.
- Covers the basics of AI and its relevance in early disease detection, different types of skin cancer and the critical need for early detection.
- Reviews various DL techniques, focusing on CNN for skin cancer classification.
- Provides step-by-step guidance on implementing AI techniques for skin cancer detection, including programming aspects.
- Includes illustrations and real-world examples of AI in action for early skin cancer detection.

The findings of this study will aid doctors in treating the disease at its onset, preventing future deterioration. This book can be referred to by professionals and researchers.

Skin Cancer Detection Using Artificial Intelligence Techniques

Parikshit N. Mahalle, Nuzhat Faiz Shaikh,
Pritibala S. Ingle and Yashwant Sudhakar Ingle

CRC Press
Taylor & Francis Group
Boca Raton London New York

CRC Press is an imprint of the
Taylor & Francis Group, an **informa** business

First edition published 2026
by CRC Press
4 Park Square, Milton Park, Abingdon, Oxon, OX14 4RN

and by CRC Press
2385 NW Executive Center Drive, Suite 320, Boca Raton FL 33431

CRC Press is an imprint of Informa UK Limited

British Library Cataloguing-in-Publication Data
A catalogue record for this book is available from the British Library

ISBN: 978-1-032-89310-5 (hbk)
ISBN: 978-1-032-89313-6 (pbk)
ISBN: 978-1-003-54215-5 (ebk)

DOI: 10.1201/9781003542155

Typeset in Times
by Newgen Publishing UK

Contents

Preface

"कर्मण्येवाधिकारस्ते मा फलेषु कदाचन।
मा कर्मफलहेतुर्भूर्मा ते संगोऽस्त्वकर्मणि॥

— *Bhagavad Gita (2:47)*

You have the right to perform your duty, but not to the fruits thereof. Let not the fruits of action be your motive, nor let your attachment be to inaction.

This timeless verse from the *Bhagavad Gita* captures the guiding spirit behind this work—a reminder to pursue knowledge and innovation with sincerity, detachment, and purpose. It is this principle that inspired our collective journey in the creation of this book.

Skin Cancer Detection Using Artificial Intelligence Techniques represents a convergence of medicine, data science, and human compassion. The book explores how artificial intelligence (AI) can serve as a transformative tool in healthcare—enabling early detection, improving diagnostic precision, and ensuring equitable access to clinical support, particularly in resource-constrained settings.

The foundation of this book lies in the **doctoral research of Dr. Yashwant Sudhakar Ingle**, which focused on developing an explainable, ethical, and efficient AI framework for automated skin cancer detection. The research was guided and enriched under the academic mentorship of **Dr. Nuzhat Faiz Shaikh**, whose expertise and continuous support shaped its scientific depth and clarity. **Dr. Parikshit N. Mahalle**, a distinguished academic leader and constant source of encouragement, provided strategic direction and scholarly guidance throughout the research and writing process. **Ms. Pritibala S. Ingle** contributed significantly through her organizational, analytical, and editorial support, ensuring the seamless compilation and refinement of the chapters.

Together, the authors have sought to combine technical rigor with social relevance—bridging AI, healthcare, and public policy into a unified, human-centered narrative. The emphasis on explainable AI, federated learning, and ethical design reflects our commitment to advancing responsible AI for real-world clinical benefit.

A comprehensive **bibliography** is included at the end of this book.

It represents the complete body of literature reviewed and consulted during the doctoral research and the preparation of this volume. While individual in-text citations are not included, the ideas, frameworks, and discussions presented throughout the chapters are deeply informed by these scholarly works.

The authors extend heartfelt gratitude to their respective institutions for their unwavering academic support:

Vishwakarma Institute of Technology (VIT), Pune;
MES Wadia College of Engineering, Wadia Campus, Pune; and
Sinhgad College of Science, Pune.

Special acknowledgment is due to the students, colleagues, and family members whose encouragement, patience, and inspiration made this intellectual endeavor possible.

May this book serve as a contribution to both science and society—reminding readers that true progress arises not merely from technology, but from purpose-driven innovation guided by empathy and ethical responsibility.

About the Authors

Parikshit N. Mahalle is a senior member of IEEE and currently serves as Professor and Dean of Academics at Vishwakarma Institute of Technology (VIT), Pune. He has previously held key roles such as Dean of Research and Development at both VIT and Vishwakarma Institute of Information Technology, as well as Head of AI and Data Science. He holds a Ph.D. from Aalborg University, Denmark, and completed postdoctoral research at CMI, Copenhagen. With 25 years of experience, he has contributed extensively through teaching, research, and academic leadership.

He has published over 440 research papers, holds 117 patents, and authored or edited 77 books with leading publishers. His research work has received significant citations across Google Scholar, Scopus, and Web of Science. He serves on editorial boards and as editor-in-chief for reputed journals. His expertise spans ML, data science, IoT, security, algorithms, and identity management.

Mahalle has guided eight Ph.D. scholars successfully and mentors several others. He has received numerous awards, including Best Faculty Award, S4DS Researcher of the Year 2023, and IEEE ICTBIG Distinguished Research Guide Award. As global academic contributor, he has delivered over 400 lectures and collaborated in 24 countries.

Nuzhat Faiz Shaikh is Professor and Head, Department of Computer Engineering, Modern Education Society's College of Engineering, Pune, India. She holds a B.E. from Cummins College of Engineering for Women, an M.E. from Pune Institute of Computer Technology, and a Ph.D. in Computer Science and Engineering from SGGSIET, Swami Ramanand Teerth Marathwada University, Nanded. With over 28 years of academic and research experience, she has published more than 100 papers in reputed journals and conferences and has authored and edited several books. Her research areas include AI, soft computing, bio-inspired optimization, and augmented and virtual reality. She serves as a reviewer for numerous reputed journals and conferences. She is a life member of CSI and ISTE and recipient of the "Educator Excellence Award 2018" by Odser Charitable Trust for her outstanding contribution to education.

Pritibala S. Ingle is Assistant Professor, Department of Computer Application, Sinhgad College of Science, Pune, India. She earned her B.Sc. and M.Sc. in Computer Science from Sant Gadge Baba Amravati University and qualified the State Eligibility Test (SET). She earned her M.C.A. and she is pursuing her Ph.D. in Computer Management at IMCC, Savitribai Phule Pune University. With over 14 years of teaching and research experience, she has published several papers in reputed journals and conferences. Her research interests include AI, data science, blockchain, and algorithms. She is actively involved in guiding undergraduate and postgraduate students in applied computer science projects and promoting the use of emerging technologies in education.

Yashwant Sudhakar Ingle is Assistant Professor, Department of Artificial Intelligence and Data Science, Pune, India. He holds a B.E. in Computer Science and Engineering from Amravati University and an M.Tech. in Computer Science and Engineering from Visvesvaraya National Institute of Technology (VNIT), Nagpur. He completed his Ph.D. in Computer Engineering at SKNCOE, Savitribai Phule Pune University with Best Paper Award at IEEE Punecon 2024. He contributes effectively in IEEE conferences as an organizing committee member, reviewer, and author. With over 15 years of academic and research experience, he has published more than 50+ research papers and 40 patents, including 10 granted in India, the USA, and the UK. He serves as a reviewer for IEEE conferences and *ASTES Journal*. He qualified GATE 2010, GATE 2020, GATE 2025 with 98, 93, 93 percentiles, respectively. His research interests include AI, soft computing, and algorithms. Mr. Ingle is a life member of ISTE, IEEE, and the VNIT Alumni Association and has received multiple awards and recognitions for his research and innovation from I2OR, IMRF, and Avishkar Foundation.

1 Skin Cancer and Causes

1.1 INTRODUCTION

In the 21st century, skin cancer has become one of the most difficult health challenges to tackle. Incidence rates are on the rise around the world, and it makes up about one-third of all diagnosed cancers globally. Skin cancer is indeed the most preventable form of cancer; however, if it is not caught in its early stages, it continues to be a major cause of morbidity and mortality. This paradox—the "disease" of commonality, yet "cured" by timely intervention—makes skin cancer a critical concern not only for clinicians, researchers, and policymakers but also for tech developers.

Skin cancer is at the very least a consequence of the skin cells' abnormal and uncontrollable growth, which is mainly the result of DNA damage. By far the single most important environmental risk factor is UV radiation, both from the sun and from artificial sources such as tanning beds. Nonetheless, UV radiation alone does not account for the entire problem. Besides, genetic susceptibility, immune suppression, exposure to chemicals, and poor living habits increase the risk for an individual. The interconnection among these factors is revealing and points to the disease's multifactorial nature that necessitates an integrated grasp of both biological processes and environmental factors.

The issue of skin cancer from public health perspective has an otherwise dismal conclusion. Countries in which the population's majority is fair-skinned, like Australia, New Zealand, and parts of Europe, have the highest incidence rates but the disease is not restricted to those areas. Cases are, in fact, increasingly observed in darker-skinned populations where clinical suspicion is lower and consequently, the diagnosis is often delayed. The trend points to the widespread importance of skin cancer prevention, detection, and treatment.

In terms of clinical practice, skin cancer is divided into the two main types of melanoma and non-melanoma skin cancers (NMSCs). Melanoma is the deadliest cancer, although it is the least prevalent among the two, because metastasis is very possible. It emerges from melanocytes, the skin's epidermal cells that produce pigment. Apart from melanomas, non-melanoma tumors are mainly made up of Basal Cell Carcinoma (BCC) and Squamous Cell Carcinoma (SCC). They are usually the least aggressive and the most common types. BCC, for example, rarely spreads but if left untreated it can lead to serious local destruction. SCC has a greater chance of spreading but is still nowhere close to melanoma in terms of death rate. Besides risk stratification, clinicians might also rely upon these categories and their subtypes for choosing the right interventions, and educating patients about preventive measures.

Histopathological biopsy has been the classic method for diagnosing skin cancer. In spite of being efficient, biopsies carry the burden of being invasive, consuming many resources, and not being a good option for screening large populations. Besides these, dermatologists also make use

DOI: 10.1201/9781003542155-1

of visual examination and dermoscopy which, while enhancing the accuracy of diagnosis, still rely entirely on the skills of the doctor. Intra-class variability (the same cancer showing very different forms in different patients) and inter-class similarity (benign lesions looking closely like malignant ones) make the diagnosis process pretty complicated. For example, a benign melanocytic nevus might look like early melanoma and thus lead to needless biopsies, anxiety for the patient, or worse—missed diagnosis. The above-mentioned limitations point out the necessity for more reliable, objective, and scalable diagnostic methods.

There is no doubt that these developments are not yet the end of the world. The major problems that hinder the clinical use of these technologies are the following: the model of explainability that does not exist, and the bias of the datasets towards certain skin colors, and the regulatory issues. However, the research that is going on, such as the use of XAI (Explanatory Artificial Intelligence) techniques, aims at reducing these problems by illustrating the predictions and thus making the doctors and patients more confident in the treatment decision.

This book, thus, occupies a position at the meeting point of clinical dermatology with artificial intelligence (AI) research. The aim of the publication is to grant the audience a well-rounded comprehension of skin cancer—the reason it occurs, what types it has, and what problems there are in diagnosing it—and of the amazing part played by AI in solving these problems. The book, by mixing up biological knowledge with technological developments, wishes to be both an aid to scientific knowledge and assistance to clinical practice.

The readers in the upcoming chapters will start off with skin cancer's medical basis, its different forms, and diagnostic difficulties, and risk factors. This background is necessary for understanding AI's role, which will be discussed further in Chapter 2. The book then transitions smoothly into a world of AI-assisted techniques, curiosity-driven experimental investigations, and real-case scenarios resulting in suggestions and forecasting of the future. Finally, the primary aim is not only to promote the academic but also to help in the practical detection and saving of lives.

1.2 GLOBAL EPIDEMIOLOGICAL BURDEN

Skin cancer is the most prevalent cancer in the world among fair-skinned people and it is steadily spreading in areas that were previously considered low risk. The World Health Organization (WHO) estimates that each year there are more than 2–3 million cases of NMSCs and 132,000 cases of melanoma diagnosed around the planet. In the leading countries like Australia and New Zealand, the annual melanoma incidence rates of over 40 cases per 100,000 people are the highest in the world. On the other hand, Asian and African countries have historically recorded low incidence rates, but the trend is changing because of the causes like urbanization, increased longevity, and exposure to lifestyle-related risks such as tanning and lack of outdoor protection.

Despite being less frequent compared to NMSC, melanoma is responsible for most of the skin cancer deaths because of its aggressive/metastatic nature. NMSC, on the other hand, is not lethal but it still poses a considerable healthcare challenge due to its high prevalence and the necessary lifelong treatment which are costly. Skin cancer incidence is expected to double by the year 2040 if no preventive measures are adopted, according to a projection.

1.2.1 Economic Costs and Healthcare Burden

The economic implications of skin cancer are striking. The annual cost of treating skin cancers in the US alone is over USD 8 billion, with almost 50% of the total being spent on melanoma treatment. The same situation is found in Europe where the demand for dermatology services, surgical interventions, and advanced therapies such as immunotherapy is also rising. The prolonged management of the disease leads to increased costs, as patients are likely to need constant check-ups, surgeries and even cosmetic reconstructions, even if the cancer is not life-threatening.

The scenario in low- and middle-income countries is different but they too experience skin cancer-related deaths due to late diagnosis, absence of treatment, and lack of access to dermatologists. In these cases, the patient generally presents with an advanced case and mortality is consequently higher. The absence of low-cost diagnostic tools and shortage of skilled personnel contribute to the inequalities in the provision of care.

1.2.2 Psychological and Social Impact

The skin cancer issue affects mainly the patients' minds, besides the clinical and financial considerations. Patients may, however, suffer through these forms of injuries in case of successful but not complete treatment. In these societies where the physical appearance is a major factor for people's self-worth and social inclusion, such visible scars can be a source of stigma, depression, and isolation. Particularly, the younger patients have to cope with the cosmetic and emotional repercussions in both the professional and personal life realms.

Besides the patients' families, public health also suffers when the emotional burden and the patient's support are divided among the health care sectors, and in this particular case, the dermatology department bears the consequences of skin cancer care. The actual struggle of health campaigns is to focus more on the psychosocial and emotional dimensions than the medical ones in order to not only develop an effective management but also bring support systems into the existing medical networks for patients and their families.

1.2.3 Geographic and Environmental Factors

The global pattern of skin cancer is not only a reflection of people's health behavior but also their geographic positioning, the weather, and the cultural practices. Equatorial residents receive the maximum exposure to sunlight and thereby the highest risk of both melanoma and NMSCs. However, paradoxically, the incidence of skin cancer is the highest among the light-skinned population in temperate or highland areas because of less pigmentation protection from the sun's rays.

The environmental factors contributing to skin cancer are mainly the depletion of the ozone layer, which has led to a greater exposure to UV radiation, and the artificial tanning habit which is at the root of the global burden. Such habits as outdoor recreation, occupational sun exposure, and tanning bed usage contribute significantly to the global burden of skin cancer. In fact, about 450,000 NMSC cases and 10,000 melanoma cases are attributed annually to the use of tanning beds in the USA, Europe, and Australia alone.

1.2.4 Disparities in Detection and Outcomes

The case of skin cancer is no different in the sense that it affects all races. However, the differences in the detection and treatment outcomes are quite pronounced, and they are the most evident when comparing different skin types. The case here is that people with darker skin are often misdiagnosed at the beginning or even later on because the doctors still think that they are "protected" against skin cancer. As melanoma develops in these areas it is often more severe and prognosis is worse. Socioeconomic factors like healthcare accessibility, education, and promotion of awareness also come into play on the outcome aspect. For instance, the rural population has less access to dermatologists and as a result they have to wait longer for doctors to diagnose and treat these cases compared to urban populations.

1.2.5 Public Health Response and Awareness

Governments and healthcare organizations have made public health campaigns focusing on prevention and early detection in the wake of the increasing disease burden. Examples of successful interventions include slogans like "Slip-Slop-Slap" in Australia and the common application of sunscreen in Western countries. Nevertheless, the world still needs to fight in unity for some time to come. The application of protective clothing, sunblock, skin self-examination, and visits to a dermatologist as a routine practice are among the few measures that are taken to lessen the disease burden.

Moreover, technology is becoming an important factor in public health strategies. Testing of mobile apps that monitor moles, teledermatology platforms supported by AI, and cloud-based screening tools are some of the new developments aimed at linking the population with specialists. These are seen as innovations with the potential of eliminating differences between regions and thus creating equal availability of diagnostic tools.

Skin cancer has a profound and diverse impact, affecting the clinical, economic, psychological, and social spheres. The increasing number of cases worldwide puts a heavy load on healthcare systems, raises costs, and diminishes the quality of life of the patients. On the one hand, developed countries deal with the economic burden and cosmetic complications, while on the other hand, developing countries suffer from late detection and high mortality rates. The gap in diagnosis between different populations is a signal for the need for global approaches and groundbreaking technologies. These elements together make it clear that skin cancer is no longer just a health care problem; it is a social issue that demands interdisciplinary solutions, where AI can be the agent of change.

1.3 SKIN CANCER TYPES

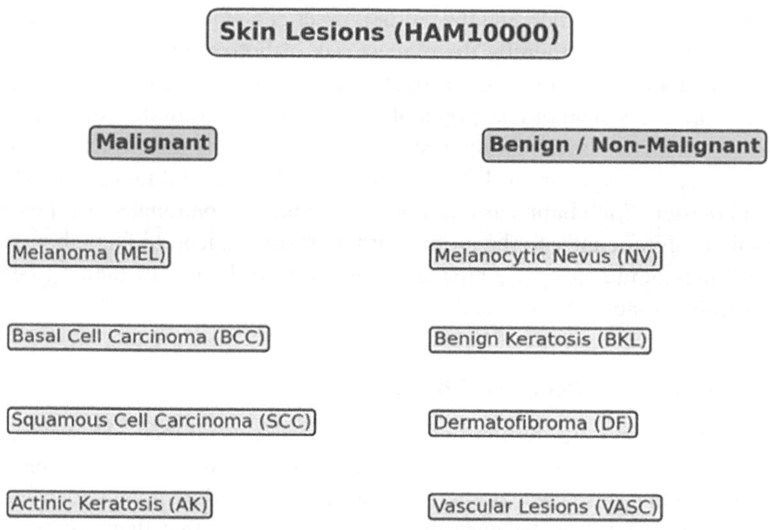

FIGURE 1.1 Classification of skin cancer.

Cancer of the skin reveals itself in a number of different clinical forms that are mainly classified into melanoma and NMSCs. Melanoma's part in the whole case picture is very small indeed, yet it still comes with the most significant death rate. NMSCs, especially BCC and SCC, are almost the same in number of cases to melanoma plus they are always considered less aggressive. Besides these, dermatology research and AI classification systems often involve the benign or premalignant lesions as well, because their resemblance to cancerous growths makes diagnosis even more difficult.

For the sake of clinical practice and computational diagnosis, eight common lesion categories are very well recognized in major datasets such as HAM10000 and ISIC:

1. Melanoma (MEL)
2. Melanocytic Nevus (NV)
3. Basal Cell Carcinoma (BCC)
4. Squamous Cell Carcinoma (SCC)
5. Actinic Keratosis (AK)
6. Benign Keratosis (BKL)
7. Dermatofibroma (DF)
8. Vascular Lesions (VASC)

Thus, these categories become the rungs of the ladder for human and AI diagnostic frameworks alike.

1.3.1 Melanoma

Melanoma is produced from melanocytes, the cells responsible for the skin color, found in the lowest layer of the epidermis. Melanoma creates only a small percentage (less than 5%) of skin cancers, but, due to its great ability to spread, it is the cause of more than 75% of skin cancer deaths.

The ABCDE rule is usually applied for the clinical identification of melanoma:

- Asymmetry: one part of the spot is different from the other.
- Border irregularity: the edges are broken up or not clearly defined.
- Color variation: many tones—brown, black, even red, blue, and white.
- Diameter: suspicious are the lesions larger than 6 mm.
- Evolving: change in size, shape, or other characteristics like itching or bleeding.

Dermoscopy increases the accuracy of diagnosis by uncovering the atypical pigment networks, irregular streaks, or blue-white veils. Noticing the disease in the early stage is vital, as the survival rate is over 90% for people with localized melanoma but it decreases rapidly once the cancer spreads.

1.3.2 Melanocytic Nevus (NV)

Melanocytic nevi, more commonly referred to as moles, represent non-cancerous growths of melanocytes. These proliferations are so frequent that nearly all kids and teenagers get them. Commonly, they manifest as well-defined, colored spots with even coloring and smooth edges.

Most of the time, nevi do not cause any problems, but there are some atypical or dysplastic nevi that could eventually turn into melanoma; thus, the monitoring becomes very important. To document the change of nevus, clinicians commonly use photography or dermoscopy. From the viewpoint of AI, the differentiation of benign nevi and the early stages of melanoma is one of the greatest challenges owing to the presence of similar visual features.

1.3.3 Basal Cell Carcinoma (BCC)

Among the various types of skin cancer, BCC takes the lead being the most common type and representing nearly 80% of the total cases of NMSCs. It originates in the basal layer of epidermal skin cells or keratinocytes and has a powerful association with prolonged exposure to the sun (UV radiation).

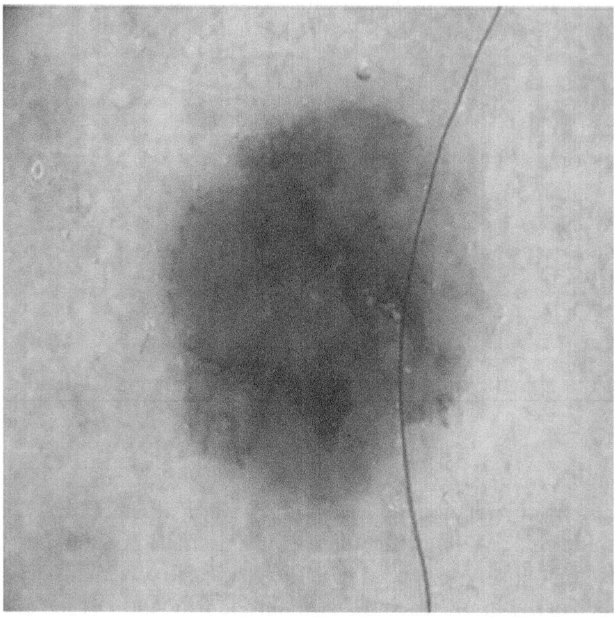

FIGURE 1.2 Dermoscopic image of melanoma.

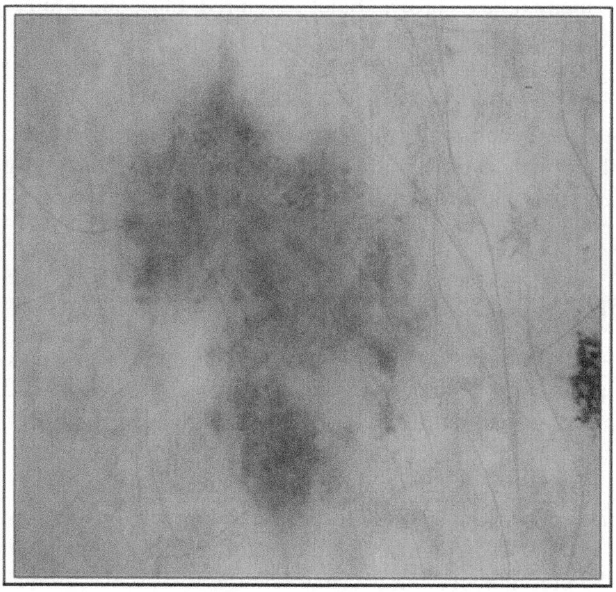

FIGURE 1.3 Dermoscopic image of melanocytic nevus (NV).

The usual manifestations of BCC are:

- Small, dome-shaped, and shiny or waxy growths, usually with small red spots (telangiectasia) that are caused by the dilatation of blood vessels.
- Slow-growing patches resembling scars with slightly blurred edges.

- Growths that can become open sores and bleed, thus the name "rodent ulcer" applied to them sometimes.

Regardless of the most recent medical developments, BCC is still one of the least likely cancers to spread but if it's left untreated, it could eventually lead to severe local destruction of the neighboring tissues invading through cartilage and bone. Fair complexion, a history of sunburns, and genetic predispositions like Gorlin syndrome are some of the factors that increase the risk.

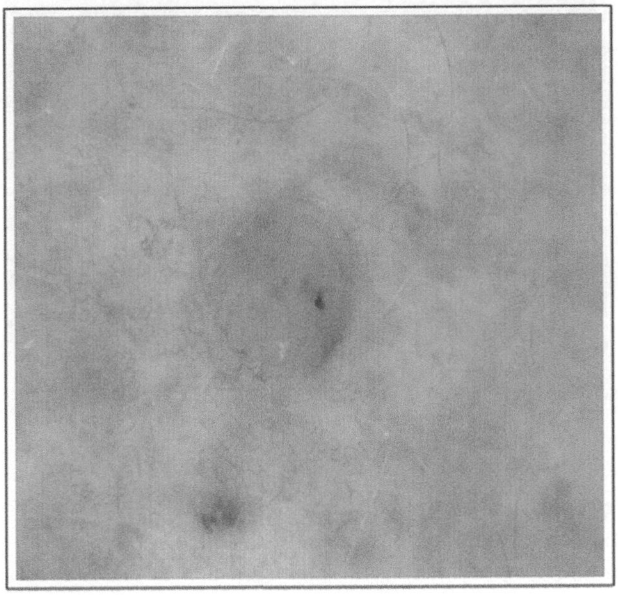

FIGURE 1.4 Dermoscopic image of basal cell carcinoma (BCC).

1.3.4 Squamous Cell Carcinoma (SCC)

SCC is of squamous keratinocyte origin and accounts for nearly 20% of NMSCs. Compared with BCC, it is more aggressive and has a greater chance of metastasizing to the lymph nodes and other organs. The clinical appearance of SCC usually comprises:

- Rough, scaly patches or plaques.
- Firm, red nodules that may develop an ulcer.
- Lesions in the areas of the body that have been most affected by the sun such as the scalp, ears, and lips.

Chronic sun exposure, immunosuppression, and chronic wounds or scars are among the risk factors for SCC. The prognosis for SCC patients is determined by the depth of invasion, tumor size, and the patient's immune system status.

1.3.5 Actinic Keratosis (AK)

Actinic keratosis, which is also called solar keratosis, is a pre-cancerous skin change that occurs as a consequence of cumulative sun exposure. It is usually regarded as the first stage of SCC in situ, meaning it can evolve into invasive SCC if not treated.
The main signs of AK are:

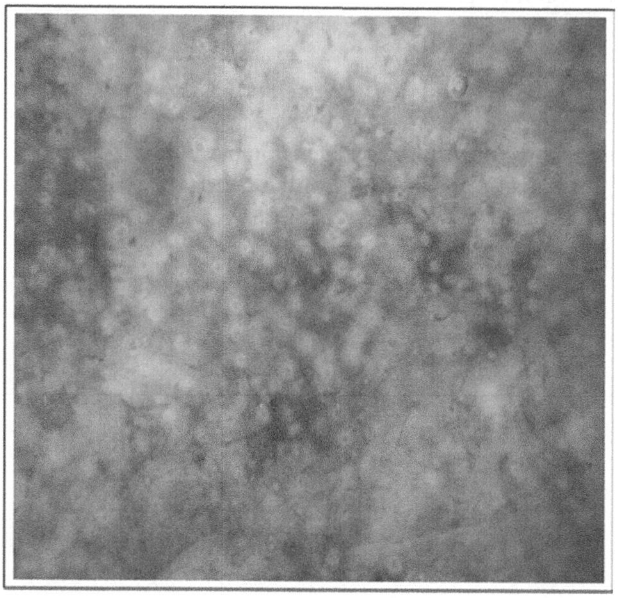

FIGURE 1.5 Dermoscopic image of squamous cell carcinoma (SCC).

- Patches that are rough, scaly, or crusty.
- Different colors such as red, brown, or even flesh-toned.
- Mainly in areas that have been exposed to the sun such as the face, ears, scalp, and hands.

Although a lot of AK lesions do not change or go away, their capacity for malignancy makes them a major target for intervention at the earliest stage. Aside from that, treatments consist of cryotherapy, topical chemotherapy (e.g., 5-fluorouracil), or photodynamic therapy.

1.3.6 Benign Keratosis (BKL)

Lesions classified as benign keratoses comprise conditions like seborrheic keratosis, solar lentigo, and lichen planus-like keratosis. Non-cancerous lesions are the ones that usually imitate melanoma because of irregular pigmentation or borders.

Seborrheic keratosis is the type that appears as "stuck-on" warty plaques having a waxy surface. Solar lentigo, on the other hand, is a skin condition linked to sun exposure and characterized by flat, pigmented spots. Despite their non-cancerous nature, these lesions still cause unnecessary biopsies most of the time because they look like melanoma in dermoscopic images.

From an AI point of view, it is vital to tell BKL apart from melanoma in order to prevent misdiagnoses and patients' anxiety.

1.3.7 Dermatofibroma (DF)

Dermatofibroma is identified as a non-cancerous fibrous tumor which generally occurs in the lower leg. It is predominantly observed in the female population and could be resulted from minor traumas like insect bites or shaving cuts.

The distinct features are:

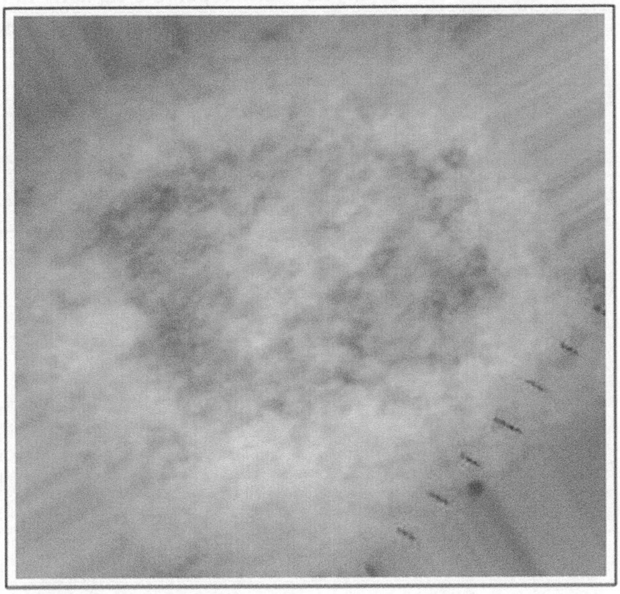

FIGURE 1.6 Dermoscopic image of actinic keratosis (AK).

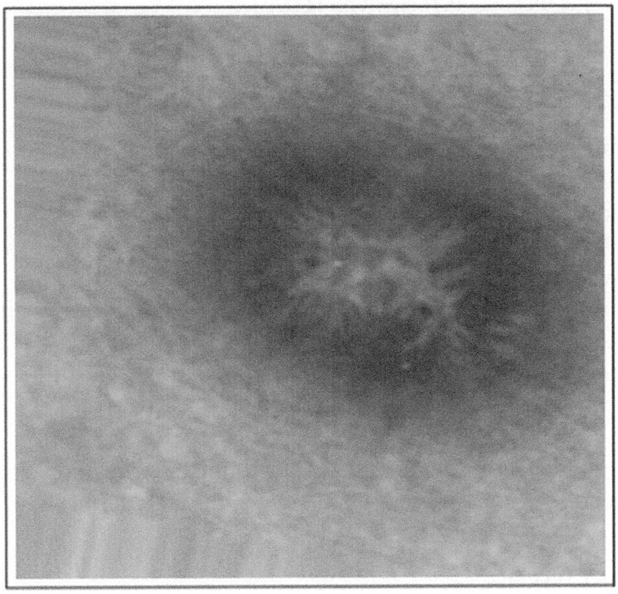

FIGURE 1.7 Dermoscopic image of benign keratosis (BKL).

- Hard, bump-like growths, most often yellowish, brownish, or reddish.
- The "dimple sign": the lesion pushes in when squeezed from side to side.
- Most of the time, it is not accompanied by any symptoms, but sometimes it may cause pain or itching.

On the other hand, DFs although non-cancerous, have developed the capacity to imitate melanoma with their color and shape, thus posing a challenge for both dermatologists and AI systems in the diagnosis.

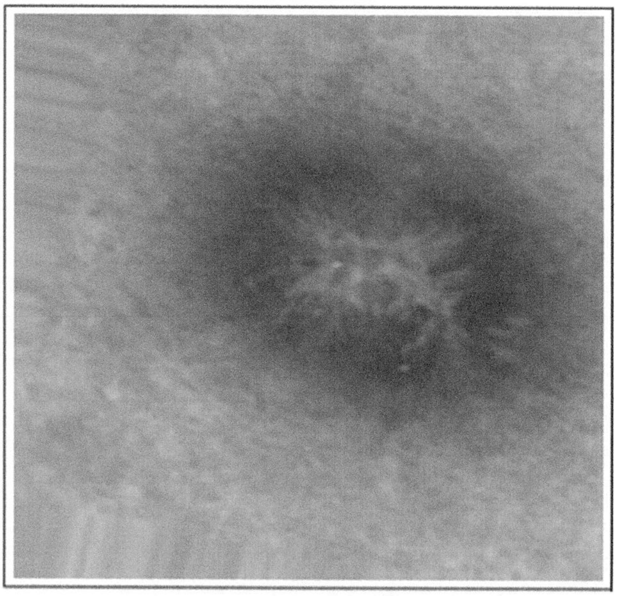

FIGURE 1.8 Dermoscopic image of dermatofibroma (DF).

1.3.8 Vascular Lesions (VASC)

VASC refer to a number of conditions that involve the abnormal production or the relaxation of blood vessels, including angiomas, hemangiomas, and pyogenic granulomas.

Clinical presentation

- Angiomas: tiny, cherry-red papules
- Hemangiomas: tumors formed at birth or in the first years of life, very often bright red ("strawberry" hemangiomas)
- Pyogenic granulomas: quickly growing red lumps that are very likely to bleed after being injured lightly.

All these lesions are non-cancerous and yet may lead to misinterpretation as cancerous tumors due to their bright colors and irregular vascular features seen through dermoscopy.

1.3.9 Comparative Overview

The various skin lesions that dermatologists encounter on a daily basis show the difficulty of diagnosing and the necessity of having strong AIs. Benign tumors frequently look like malignant tumors, and the latter, in turn, may present very different appearances according to the age of the patient, the type of skin, and the site of lesion.

In conclusion:

- Melanoma has the highest mortality rate but is also the least common type.
- BCC is the most common type of skin cancer but is the least aggressive.

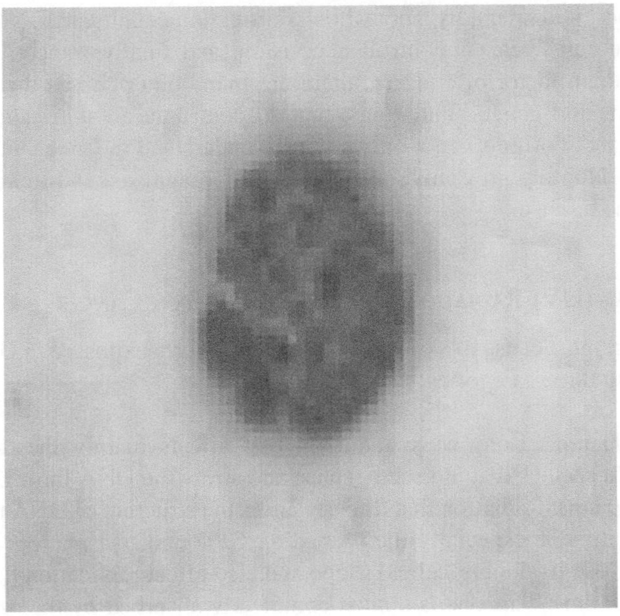

FIGURE 1.9 Dermoscopic image of vascular lesion (VASC).

- SCC is between the two with a considerable risk of spreading.
- AK, BKL, DF, and VASC are among the skin conditions that can be confused with cancer producing a challenging diagnostic situation.

TABLE 1.1
Classification of Skin Cancer Lesions

Skin Lesion Type	Category	Nature
Melanoma	Melanoma	Malignant
Melanocytic Nevus (NV)	Melanoma-related	Benign
Basal Cell Carcinoma (BCC)	Non-Melanoma	Malignant
Actinic Keratosis (AK)	Non-Melanoma	Pre-malignant
Benign Keratosis (BKL)	Non-Melanoma	Benign
Dermatofibroma (DF)	Non-Melanoma	Benign
Vascular Lesion (VASC)	Non-Melanoma	Benign
Squamous Cell Carcinoma (SCC)	Non-Melanoma	Malignant

Skin cancer and lesions of the skin, their different types, and understanding skin cancer pathology are the preconditions for accurate diagnosis and proper treatments. The eight lesion categories included in the discussion are the basis for modern dermatological image datasets and at the same time, the most difficult challenge for the classification systems worked out by AI. It is systematic distinction between these lesion types that researchers and clinicians are aiming at in order to reduce diagnostic errors, avoid unnecessary biopsies, and improve patient outcomes.

1.4 SKIN CANCER ORIGIN

The creation of skin cancer is a complicated process that consists of multiple steps and is primarily dependent on the interplay among genetic predisposition, environmental factors, and lifestyle choices. The issue is fundamentally about how skin cells accumulate DNA damage, leading to misregulation of the cell cycle, uncontrolled division, and finally, cancer. Although tanning by sunlight is still the main factor of concern, there are many other causes that are indirect, such as chemical carcinogens and genetic mutations, that all contribute to skin cancer development. The knowledge of skin cancer origins is not only a way to understand the mechanisms involved but also provides a basis for adopting preventive measures, early diagnosis, and treatment options that are less effective than the disease.

1.4.1 Ultraviolet (UV) Radiation and the Risk of Skin Cancer

The very first and foremost cause of skin cancer is the long-term exposure to UV radiation. UV radiation is classified into three categories:

- UVA (320–400 nm): Long-wave radiation that affects mainly the dermis layer, creating reactive oxygen species that indirectly cause and stress the DNA through oxidation.
- UVB (280–320 nm): Radiation that directly alters the structure of DNA through the formation of pyrimidine dimers, especially the bicreating CPD and 6–4 photoproducts. These lesions cause DNA to lose its double-helical shape and also affect replication poorly.
- UVC (100–280 nm): This one is almost completely absorbed by the ozone layer and is thus not a major factor in the natural environment.

The human body possesses intrinsic repair systems, one of which is the nucleotide excision repair (NER), available for mending UV-damaged DNA. In large doses, however, UV radiation may cause an irreversible change in the genes controlling the repair systems. For instance:

- Mutations in p53, which is a tumor suppressor gene, happen frequently in squamous cell carcinoma.
- Most often, PTCH1 gene alterations are seen in basal cell carcinoma, and so on.
- BRAF and NRAS oncogenes are mutated and thus lead to the development of melanoma.
- The occurrence of the aforementioned cases of nonrepair is therefore a significant carcinogenic event.

1.4.2 Genetic Predisposition

Inheriting genetic abnormalities can make a person more exposed to getting skin cancer regardless of the presence of environmental factors; still the main reason for getting skin cancer remains UV radiation. For instance:

- Mutations in CDKN2A and CDK4, which control the cell cycle, are frequently responsible for familial melanoma.
- Xeroderma pigmentosum (XP), which is a very rare genetic condition, leads to the inability to repair the DNA damage caused by the sun. Such individuals are at extreme risk of developing melanoma and NMSC at an early age.
- Gorlin syndrome (nevoid basal cell carcinoma syndrome), which is a result of PTCH1 mutations, is characterized by the appearance of numerous BCCs over one's lifetime.

Genetic syndromes like the ones mentioned earlier are evidence of how environmental exposure is intensified by the intrinsic genetic vulnerability.

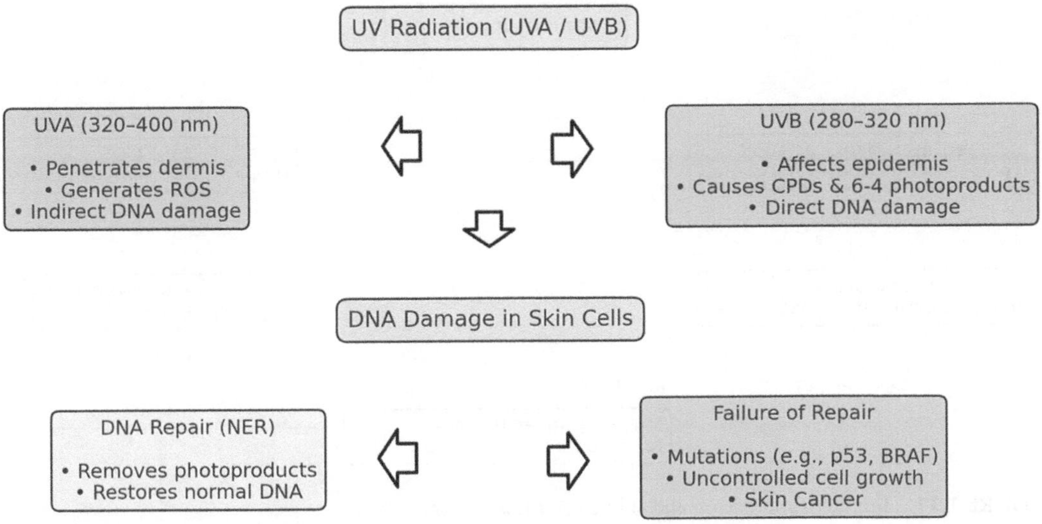

FIGURE 1.10 Mechanism of UV radiation-induced DNA damage in skin cells.

1.4.3 Immunosuppression and Infection

A healthy immune system is central to the process of recognizing and getting rid of abnormal cells before they turn into cancer. Due to the fact that immunosuppression—whether it happens due to medical treatment or condition—removes the safety net, the situation becomes more severe.

- Those who have undergone organ transplants and are using immunosuppressant drugs for a long time are at a particularly high risk for developing skin cancer, especially SCC. In fact, those who have had a transplant can have an incidence of SCC that is up to 65 times higher than that of the general population.
- People with HIV and those suffering from chronic immunosuppressive conditions are similarly susceptible to skin cancer.
- Certain viral infections play an indirect role: for example, human papillomavirus (HPV) has been linked to the development of SCC in patients with a weakened immune system.

1.4.4 Chemical and Occupational Exposures

Exposure to carcinogenic substances can initiate or accelerate skin cancer development. Historically, occupational exposures have played a major role:

- Arsenic, found in contaminated water or used in some pesticides, is a known risk factor for both SCC and BCC.
- Polycyclic aromatic hydrocarbons (PAHs), encountered by chimney sweeps, tar workers, and industrial employees, have long been associated with skin cancer.
- Chronic exposure to ionizing radiation, such as in medical workers or patients receiving radiotherapy, also increases risk.

Modern occupational health measures have reduced these risks in developed countries, but they remain significant in low-resource settings.

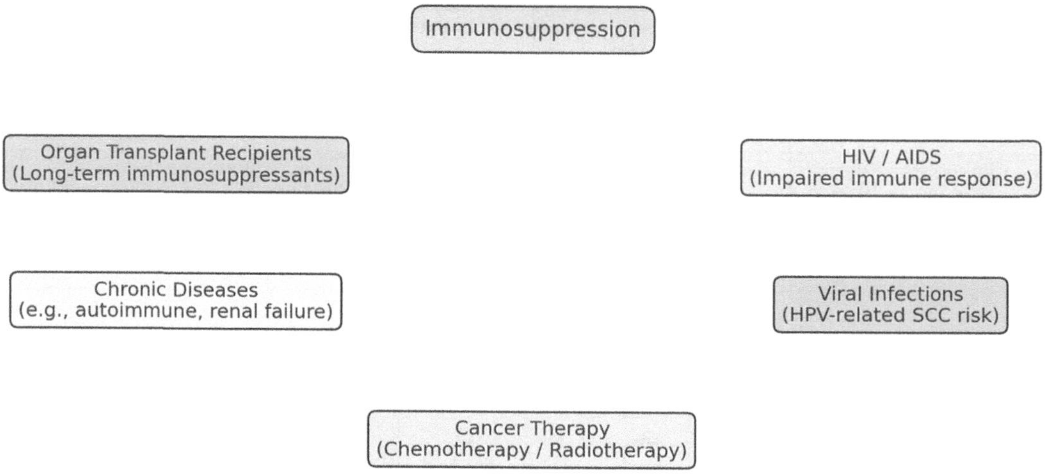

FIGURE 1.11 Immunosuppression and skin cancer risk factors.

1.4.5 Chronic Inflammation and Wounds

Persistent inflammation or scar tissue can be a cause of cancer. One such example is Marjolin's ulcer, where cancerous tissues invade and grow within previously damaged areas of the body, such as chronic and inflamed burns, scarred wounds, or spots that endure constant trauma. The process of turning over cells over and over due to the chronic inflammatory environment makes it easy for the DNA to get mutated and the cell to get transformed into a malignant one.

1.4.6 Lifestyle and Behavioral Factors

Certain lifestyle habits are a major contributing factor to skin cancer risk:

- Artificial tanning machines: These are known as Group 1 carcinogens by the International Agency for Research on Cancer (IARC), thus tanning beds are a major contributor to melanoma and NMSC risk, especially among those who use it before turning 30.
- Sun exposure during outdoor activities without protection: Such recreational activities as going to the beach, mountain climbing, or playing sports outdoors without sufficient sunscreen lead to a great accumulation of UV damage.
- Smoking: Smoking is mainly responsible for lung cancer, but it has also been linked with SCC possibly because of its immunosuppressive and DNA-damaging effects.

The public health campaigns are increasingly focusing on these behaviors by telling people to be more cautious, wear protective clothing, and avoid tanning devices.

1.4.7 Molecular Pathogenesis

The transition of skin from normal to cancerous state is accompanied by a series of molecular changes:

1. Initiation: UV or chemical exposure causes DNA damage that results in mutations.
2. Promotion: Non-normal cells get an advantage in growing and multiplying.

3. Progression: More mutations make the cells invasive and develop their own blood supply and metastasize.

The main molecular pathways are:

- Hedgehog signaling pathway involved in BCC.
- MAPK pathway (BRAF, NRAS) in melanoma.
- P53 mutations associated with SCC.

Understanding these pathways has opened doors to targeted therapies, such as BRAF inhibitors for melanoma and hedgehog pathway inhibitors for BCC.

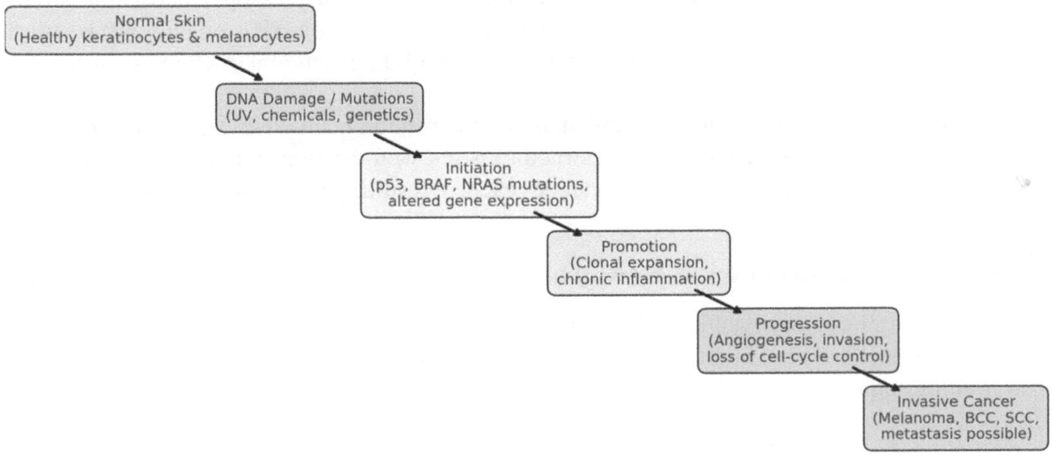

FIGURE 1.12 Multistep molecular progression from normal skin to invasive cancer.

The origins of skin cancer are multifactorial, involving a dynamic interplay of UV radiation, genetic predispositions, immune surveillance, chemical exposures, and lifestyle choices. While UV radiation remains the most significant factor, hereditary syndromes and immunosuppression highlight the importance of genetic and systemic contributors. Modern molecular biology has elucidated key signaling pathways that not only clarify the mechanisms of carcinogenesis but also provide therapeutic targets. By understanding these origins, clinicians and researchers can better strategize prevention, develop targeted therapies, and design AI-based systems that incorporate risk factors beyond visual image analysis.

1.5 MEDICAL OVERVIEW OF SKIN CANCER AND DIAGNOSTIC DIFFICULTIES

Skin cancer is different from all other types of cancer in humans because it appears in the most visible organ—the skin. The visibility of skin cancer provides the chance for early detection, but the diagnostics continue to provide challenges which seem to be even more aggravated than before. Even the smallest differences in the morphology of the lesions and the scarcity of trained specialists all contribute to the difficulties in managing and treating skin cancer which now requires the precision of science and the allocation of practical resources. Diagnostics and their limitations have been described in this section together with the complications that create a barrier to accurate and timely identification.

1.5.1 Traditional Diagnostic Pathway

The typical method used for skin cancer diagnosis consists of a sequence of steps as follows:

1. Clinical Examination: Dermatologists check the wounds by visual inspection using the naked eye. The main warning signs of skin cancers are asymmetry, irregular borders, color variation, and ulceration.
2. Dermoscopy: The handheld dermatoscope that is used magnifies and illuminates the skin lesions, and the subsurface patterns that are not visible to the naked eye get revealed. Dermoscopy has considerably improved the accuracy of diagnosis. However, in most situations the final decision on whether the lesion is malignant or not will depend upon the expertise of the clinician.
3. Histopathological Biopsy: If the lesion seems to be suspicious, a biopsy is carried out. The tissue is taken out, processed, and examined under a microscope. Histopathology is still the golden standard, and it gives the final word in terms of diagnosis and grading of cancer.

Even though this method is effective, still it is time-consuming, invasive, and there are various access barriers. In areas where health infrastructure is not well developed, patients have to endure long waits before histopathology services can be reached, resulting in late detection of the disease.

1.5.2 Diagnostic Accuracy and Limitations

Diagnosis is still not great even in high-resource settings. Dermatologists' accuracy for melanoma diagnosis has been reported in different studies to be between 60% and 80%. This range depends on their training and experience. The problem with these lesions is the overlap:

- Inter-class similarity: Small benign melanocytic nevi frequently mimic early-stage melanoma.
- Intra-class variability: One type of cancer may show different symptoms depending on skin color of the patient, lesion site, and stage of the disease.
- Atypical presentations: Tumors like pigmented BCC or amelanotic melanoma do not present with typical features and are easily overlooked.

These uncertainties in the diagnosis can result in both false positives (which are unnecessary biopsies and patient anxiety) and negatives (missed malignancies with potentially fatal outcomes).

1.5.3 Imaging Modalities in Dermatology

Dermoscopy is accompanied by various imaging technologies to enhance the accuracy of diagnosis:

- Confocal Laser Scanning Microscopy (CLSM): It gives almost histological resolution images of skin layers in living patients.
- Optical Coherence Tomography (OCT): It generates cross-sectional images that are beneficial in determining lesion depth and margins.
- Histopathological Imaging: The microscopic examination of stained tissue samples from excisional biopsies is still the most reliable method.
- Hyperspectral Imaging (HSI): It collects the spectral signatures of lesions across different wavelengths, thus providing their biochemical and structural characterization.
- Total Body Photography (TBP): It is applied to monitor the changes of numerous moles over time in patients who are at risk.

Each of these methods has its own set of benefits and also faces the challenges of being costly, having limited availability, and requiring a lot of time for the clinician to master.

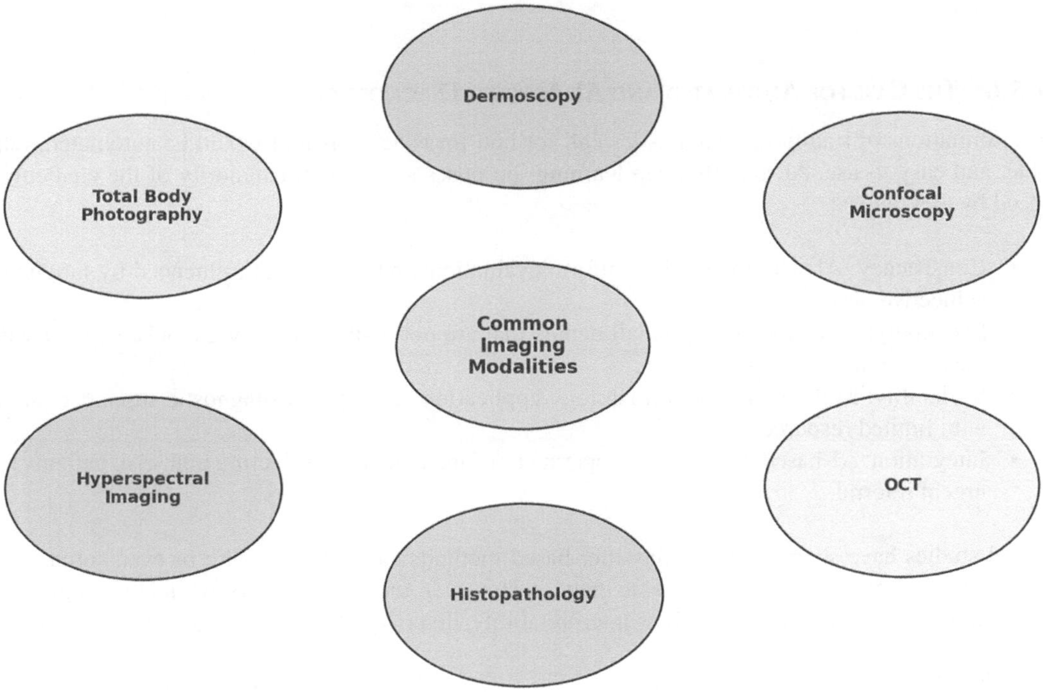

FIGURE 1.13 Common imaging modalities used in skin cancer detection.

1.5.4 Accessibility and Resource Barriers

Access to specialized dermatology services is still not the same all over the world. For instance, in low- and middle-income countries, there are very few dermatologists and they are mainly found in urban centers. Rural people have to face both geographic and financial obstacles, which results in the diagnoses being made only when cancers have reached advanced stages. Even in very well-off countries, a lot of patients are referred to specialists, which can mean a long wait before being seen by one.

In addition, biopsies and sophisticated imaging procedures require a lot of resources. As a result, patients in different parts of the world receive healthcare services on an unequal basis, and among them, the people living in the underserved regions suffer the most as they have to cope with late diagnoses and consequently, the worst outcomes.

1.5.5 Psychological and Clinical Consequences of Delayed or Inaccurate Diagnosis

The effects of diagnostic disputes are not limited to medical outcomes. A positive cancer diagnosis might lead to a patient being sent for an unnecessary biopsy. Although these are invasive, they are also costly and very disturbing mentally for the patients. The same thing will happen with the confusion of the patients caused by repeated biopsies, which they may get and fear because of the scarring and aesthetic issues. That is the case with false negatives too, but it is even worse: the death of a melanoma patient might be caused by a diagnosed tumor allowed to grow untruncated by the cancerous cells, and thus, the chance of survival has been decreased greatly.

Patients usually feel anxious during the wait for biopsy results, which can take days to weeks. In addition, and even worse, a person's self-esteem, social interactions, and general quality of life may suffer if he or she is disfigured as a result of large excisions or reconstructive surgery following late detection.

1.5.6 The Case for Automated and AI-Assisted Diagnostics

The limitations of traditional diagnostics call for non-invasive tools that would be automated, reliable, and easy to use. AI, mainly deep learning, proposes solutions for majority of the challenges faced by these areas:

- Consistency: Algorithms render uniform evaluations, which are not influenced by fatigue or subjective bias.
- Sensitivity: AI can spot very small details that are not visible even by the naked eye or with the help of dermoscopy.
- Scalability: Mobile and teledermatology applications can extend diagnostic support to areas with limited resources.
- Integration: AI-based systems may operate as triage machines, selecting high-risk patients for urgent referral.

Initial studies have shown that AI classifier-based methods can compare with or even surpass the accuracy of dermatologists in diagnostic matters. However, the integration of AI in clinical practice will require overcoming issues such as interpretability, diversity of datasets, and ethical dilemmas.

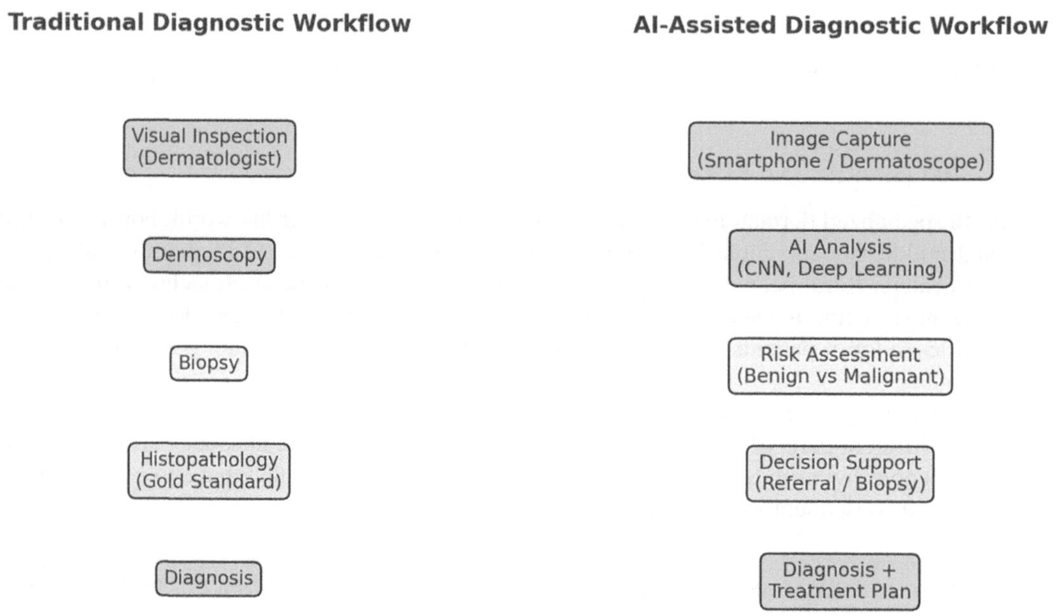

FIGURE 1.14 Comparison of traditional diagnostic workflow vs. AI-assisted workflow.

The medical perspective of skin cancer diagnosis unveils a paradox: even though the disease is visible and preventable, its accurate detection is still a big challenge. The traditional methods: clinical inspection, dermatoscopy, and biopsy are necessary but they all have their own drawbacks. For instance, these methods are subjective, invasive, and not easily accessible. The use of advanced imaging techniques, on the other hand, increases sensitivity but still they are very expensive and not available in many areas. The diagnostic discrepancies underline the urgent demand for AI-powered systems, which are well-considered for their consistency, scalability, and improvement in accuracy. Thus, the combination of traditional medicine with technology represents the way to lessen the global burden of skin cancer.

1.6 SKIN CANCER THEORETICAL BACKGROUND

It is vital to have a theoretical basis of skin biology and carcinogenesis first to understand the mechanisms, risk factors, and diagnostic difficulties of skin cancer. Theoretical background comprises the skin's structure, the cellular origins of cancer, the transition from healthy tissue to invasive cancer, and the biological markers used in diagnosis and prognosis. This information not only delineates the medical context of skin cancer but also assists in the creation of AI-based detection systems that rely on recognizing the structural and morphological patterns.

1.6.1 Anatomy and Structure of Human Skin

The skin is the largest organ of the body, covering about 1.5–2 square meters in adults, and being responsible for nearly 15% of the weight of the body. Along with the above-mentioned, it also acts as a barrier against all types of injuries, microorganisms, UV rays, and water loss. It is made up of three main layers:

1. Epidermis
    - The uppermost layer of the skin.
    - Mostly made up of keratinocytes that give the skin strength and the ability to resist penetration.
    - Home to melanocytes (cells that produce pigment), Merkel cells (touch receptors), and Langerhans cells (immune monitoring).
    - A great number of skin cancers, including BCC, SCC, and melanoma, arise from the basal layer (stratum basale).
2. Dermis
    - Located under the epidermis.
    - Formed by connective tissue with collagen, elastin fibers, and a matrix supplied with blood vessels, lymphatics, and nerves.
    - Takes care of the epidermis by giving it structural support, maintaining its temperature, and supplying it with nutrients.
3. Hypodermis (Subcutaneous tissue)
    - Last layer, which is largely made of fat tissue.
    - Functions as an insulator, a source of energy, and as a protective layer for the organs underneath.

1.6.2 Cellular Origins of Skin Cancer

Skin cancer is a term that encompasses various types of abscesses and tumors that develop in the skin through different cell types:

- Melanoma: It is a tumor with the origin from the melanocytes found in the basal layer of the epidermis.
- BCC: It is a tumor with the origin from basal keratinocytes.
- SCC: It is a tumor with its origin from the squamous keratinocytes located in the upper epidermal layer.

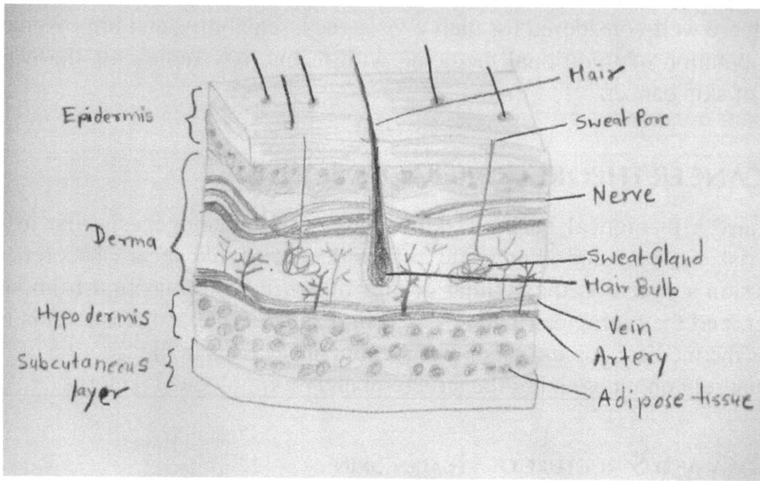

FIGURE 1.15 Anatomy of human skin showing epidermis, dermis, and hypodermis.

- AK: It is a precancerous condition that is considered as the first stage of SCC.
- Other lesions (DF, BKL, VASC): They are the lesions that have their origin related to fibroblasts, keratinocytes, or vascular endothelial cells based on the type of lesion.

Cancer type is defined with histological and molecular characteristics that are different from each other but the commonality between them is the fact that all of them are due to genetic mutations leading to uncontrolled cell proliferation.

1.6.3 Multistep Carcinogenesis

The process of turning normal skin into malignant cancer is a multistep one:

1. Initiation:
   - Skin DNA is damaged by UV irradiation, chemicals, or inherited genetic factors.
   - The mutations in tumor suppressor (e.g., p53) and oncogenes (e.g., BRAF, NRAS) genes slowly accumulate.
2. Promotion:
   - The cells that have suffered damage become the ones that can divide more rapidly.
   - The surroundings contribute to this abnormal growth by providing factors like chronic inflammation and immunosuppression.
3. Progression:
   - The malignant cells become capable of invading the neighboring tissues, new blood vessel formation occurs, and the possibility of scattered tumor cells exploiting distant sites is created.

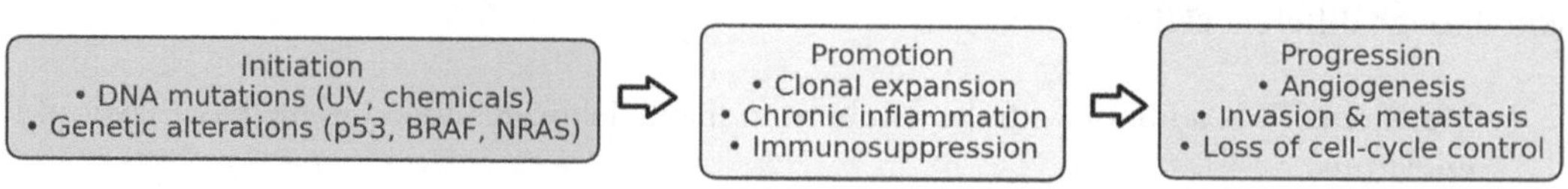

FIGURE 1.16 Multistep process of carcinogenesis: initiation, promotion, progression.

1.6.4 Molecular Pathways in Skin Cancer

One of the most important things revealed by recent molecular biology techniques is that there are several important signaling pathways that lead to skin cancer:

- Hedgehog pathway: BCC shows abnormal activity in this pathway as a general characteristic; vismodegib is a type of targeted therapy that takes advantage of this pathway.
- MAPK (Mitogen-Activated Protein Kinase) pathway: This pathway is activated in melanoma because of mutations in BRAF and NRAS, which causes to uncontrolled cell division.
- P53 pathway: Non-functioning of the tumor suppressor p53 is highly correlated with SCC.

Molecular revelations are essential not only for knowing the disease progression but also for creating targeted therapies which in turn will result in better treatment outcomes for the patients.

1.6.5 Biomarkers of Skin Cancer

Biomarkers play the role of measurable signs of disease presence, progression, or therapeutic response. A few examples of the most common biomarkers studied in skin cancer are as follows:

- S100, HMB-45, and Melan-A: Immunohistochemical markers for melanomas.
- Ki-67: Proliferation marker indicating how aggressive the tumor is.
- P16INK4a: Often altered in melanoma and linked to the genetic predisposition.
- VEGF (Vascular Endothelial Growth Factor): Associated with the blood supply formation in the aggressive lesions.

AI systems that are able to learn from histopathological images are increasingly using such biomarker correlations, establishing a connection between microscopic structures and molecular profiles.

1.6.6 Clinical Staging and Prognostic Models

The clinical outcome of skin cancer mainly relies on its stage at the time of diagnosis. The TNM (Tumor, Node, Metastasis) classification is a standard system of staging that among other things aids in disease progression assessment. For instance:

- T (Tumor): Size and depth of invasion.
- N (Node): Involvement of the nearest lymph nodes.
- M (Metastasis): Spread to distant organs or sites.

In the case of melanoma, besides the tumor thickness (Breslow) and ulceration, these factors strongly dictate the prognosis. If diagnosed early when the lesions are still thin and localized, the patients have over 90% chance of surviving; on the other hand, the chances of survival of patients with metastatic melanoma are less than 20%.

1.6.7 Theoretical Context for AI Integration

Theoretical comprehension of skin cancer biology is the substrate of the AI-based diagnostic tools. Lesion shape, the histological characteristics of the epidermis and dermis, and the multistep carcinogenesis pathways can all be visualized in dermoscopic or histopathological images, where they are the most visible. AI systems, especially convolutional neural networks (CNNs), are intended to detect these fine features, which are frequently beyond the capability of a human eye. By relating the biological processes and the digital image attributes, AI not only provides a theoretical comprehension but also an access to practical diagnostic applications through this interdisciplinary aspect.

At the basis of the skin cancer hypothesis lies the anatomy of the skin, the cells from which the cancer originates and the molecular pathways leading to the development of the malignancy. The knowledge about biomarkers, staging, and progression not only supports clinical practice but also helps in designing AI-based diagnostic systems. If the computational methods are rooted in biological concepts, then the researchers and the clinicians can make sure that the AI solution is both biologically interpretable and clinically relevant.

1.7 SUMMARY

Skin cancer is increasingly seen as a public health issue that not only mixes biological aspect but also brings along social, economic, and technological factors. The current chapter has opened up the topic of the disease in a broad manner, which will continue with the AI in skin cancer detection. By discussing the causes, types, diagnostic barriers, and theoretical background, we have prepared the ground to alert the need for technological innovations in this field.

1.7.1 Recap of Major Insights

1. Prevalence and Significance
   Worldwide skin cancer is one of the most widespread types of cancer, and both melanoma and non-melanoma types are the main contributors to the high mortality rate. And, although it is highly visible and almost always preventable, its incidence globally is getting higher and higher due to the various factors, such as UV exposure, lifestyle habits, and environmental changes, including ozone layer depletion, etc.
2. Impact and Burden
   In addition to the medical burden, the disease also imposes economic and psychological burdens on society. Healthcare systems have to spend billions of dollars just to treat the disease, while patients go through and suffer from not only disfigurement but also anxiety and stigma associated with the disease. Lack of access to early detection in underserved areas increases these burdens.
3. Types and Complexity
   The clinical range of skin cancer comprises melanoma, BCC, SCC, and their related benign or pre-malignant lesions, for example, AK, BKL, DF, and VASC. The overlapping nature of these lesion types, as they frequently resemble each other, breathes life into the diagnostic difficulties that even skilled professionals might face.
4. Origins and Pathogenesis
   Skin cancer develops through a complex interaction of UV radiation, genetics, immunosuppression, chemical exposure, and chronic inflammation. The hype on the molecular level is generated by the alteration of the genes like p53, BRAF, NRAS, CDKN2A, and PTCH1 that power the unregulated growth and spread of the tumor. The concept of multistep carcinogenesis—transition through initiation, promotion, and progression—helps to trace the course of the disease.
5. Diagnostic Challenges
   Histopathology, being the gold standard, is a reliable method, but at the same time it is an invasive and resource-consuming one. Clinical examination and dermoscopy are the two methods that improve the detection, but they also have the limit of being subjective and dependent on the expertise of the person operating them. Advanced imaging modalities like OCT, CLSM, and HSI do give valuable insights; however, they are still expensive and not many can have

access to them. Variability within and between classes of diagnosis complicates visual diagnostics, thus leading to false positives and negatives.

6. Theoretical Framework for AI
   Skin anatomy, lesion morphology, pathways of carcinogenesis, and biomarkers are the factors that give a theoretical basis for computational analysis. The biological structures and processes are represented by the visual patterns in both dermoscopic and histopathological images. AI, more specifically deep learning models, is able to detect such patterns with the help of large datasets, thus providing the advantages of consistency, reproducibility, and the possibility of early intervention.

1.7.2 Transition to AI and Technology

The current diagnostic methods have numerous drawbacks and this situation is calling for innovation. Large-scale datasets' AI systems can reach diagnostic accuracies similar to or even better than those of skin doctors. What is more, these systems will be able to make it easier for even those areas with limited resources to get diagnostic support, where there is lack of dermatology knowledge. The use of AI in teledermatology and mobile technologies is a clear indication of the fact that it can make skin cancer detection more accessible to all.

On the other hand, the future of AI is still uncertain as there are drawbacks like bias in datasets, hard-to-read models, and tough-to-get approvals. Working collaboratively by computer scientists, dermatologists, policymakers, and ethicists. will help to overcome these challenges.

1.7.3 Concluding Perspective

The discussion in this chapter has demonstrated that skin cancer is not only a biological disease but a multifaceted social problem—one that encompasses prevention measures, healthcare provision, psychological assistance, and global justice. The points made here, to a large extent, explain the reason why the convergence of dermatology and AI is such an exciting frontier.
The structure of the following chapters in this book will be:

- The first chapter will walk us through the tools, technologies, and AI methods in the area of medical imaging.
- The second chapter will analyze the uses of AI in skin cancer detection, considering both public health and practical application viewpoints.
- The third chapter will provide us with experimentations and results in AI methods comparisons revealing the highs and lows of each method.
- The fourth chapter will review the solutions, recommendations, and specific cases.
- The last chapter will give a bird's-eye view of the research outcomes and future research and application directions.

By linking biological theory with technological innovation, this book seeks to demonstrate how AI can transform skin cancer detection into a faster, more accurate, and more accessible process, ultimately saving lives and reducing global disease burden.

2 Artificial Intelligence Tools and Technology

2.1 ARTIFICIAL INTELLIGENCE: AN OVERVIEW

The journey of artificial intelligence (AI) has been nothing short of remarkable. Initially, AI was a specialty area of computer science, but it gradually turned out to be the most powerful technology that could change the whole human world. To put it simply, AI is about designing computer programs that can handle the activities previously thought only possible for humans like solving problems, reasoning, learning, and perceiving. In healthcare, AI is seen as a pioneer of event, inputting new ideas to old problems and offering ways out in areas like diagnosis, treatment planning, patient monitoring, and drug discovery. In the case of dermatology, AI is expected to contribute to the better detection of skin cancer at an early stage by solving the weaknesses that are inherent in traditional diagnostics.

2.1.1 Historical Context and Evolution of AI

The idea of machine performing human thinking processes can be dated back to the 1950s when key figures like Alan Turing set up the groundwork for theoretical AI. The first AI approach that got research attention was based on the manipulations of symbols and the use of the so-called rule-based systems. Here, knowledge was structured into rules and then the inference engines would carry out the reasoning processes. These systems indeed exhibited capability in limited contexts, but they were not able to scale or adapt to the complexities of real-world problems.

The 1980s were the decade when machine learning (ML) came to prominence, an entire shift that highlighted the superiority of data-driven models over the reasoning based on rules. ML systems, instead of having knowledge programmed into them, went through the process of learning with the help of examples making it possible for them to generalize from the data. Among the classical ML techniques, decision trees, support vector machines, and random forests were quite effective for the structured data analysis; however, they could not cope with unstructured inputs like pictures, speech, or video.

The latest change has been brought about by deep learning (DL), which is a branch of machine learning that is based on the human brain's architecture and functioning. DL is particularly identified with Convolutional Neural Networks (CNNs) and these models have pushed the performance in image recognition, natural language processing (NLP), and speech recognition to unprecedented levels. In the case of dermatology, CNNs are the ones who take care of the tedious job of picking out the finest details from dermoscopic or histological images that even the most skilled dermatologists may find hard to appreciate.

DOI: 10.1201/9781003542155-2

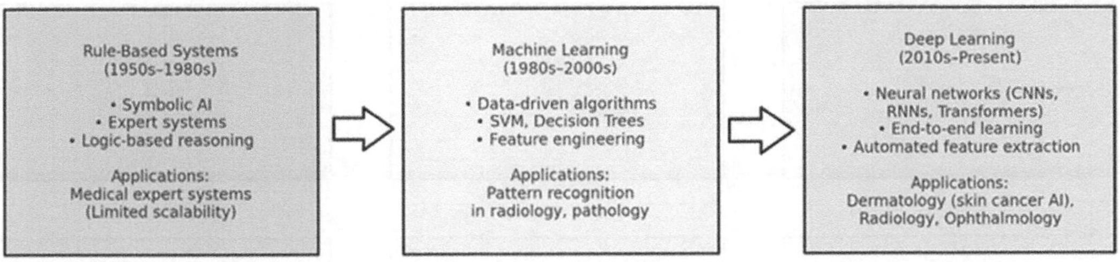

FIGURE 2.1 Evolution of AI from rule-based systems to machine learning to deep learning, with applications in healthcare.

2.1.2 Key Concepts in AI

AI is a broad field which has several subfields that are contributing to the medical applications in different ways:

- ML: Algorithms are being created to automatically get better with experience. In skin cancer detection, ML classifiers such as support vector machines or random forests can tell apart benign and malignant lesions when trained on features that are hand-crafted.
- DL: Neural networks with several layers are used to learn feature representations in a hierarchy. CNNs are the backbone of image-based diagnostics and are superior to traditional ML in skin cancer classification.
- Computer Vision: An area in AI that empowers machines to comprehend and evaluate visual data. It is in dermatology where computer vision is used in dermoscopy, clinical images, and histopathological slides.
- NLP: NLP is less related to dermatology imaging, but it does help in extracting information from electronic health records (EHRs) and linking diagnostic predictions with patient history.

All these components are cooperating and thus, they are able to produce systems which are fully capable of diagnostic support through the whole process.

2.1.3 AI in Healthcare

- The application of AI in healthcare is very diverse and covers many areas:
- Radiology: The automated detection of lung nodules, bone fractures, and brain hemorrhages.
- Pathology: Digital pathology reinforced by AI enhances cancer grading and prognosis prediction.
- Ophthalmology: AI systems can identify diabetic retinopathy and glaucoma by analyzing fundus images.
- Cardiology: Algorithms deduce arrhythmias and cardiovascular risk factors from ECGs.

Dermatology has joined this transformation more recently, with the abundance of image-based data making it particularly suitable for AI-driven solutions. Skin lesion classification, severity scoring, and risk prediction are among the most promising applications.

2.1.4 AI in Dermatology

The contribution of AI to dermatology is enormous as the dermatological field is a visual one. Diagnosis is based purely on the identification of skin lesions' patterns, colors, textures, and

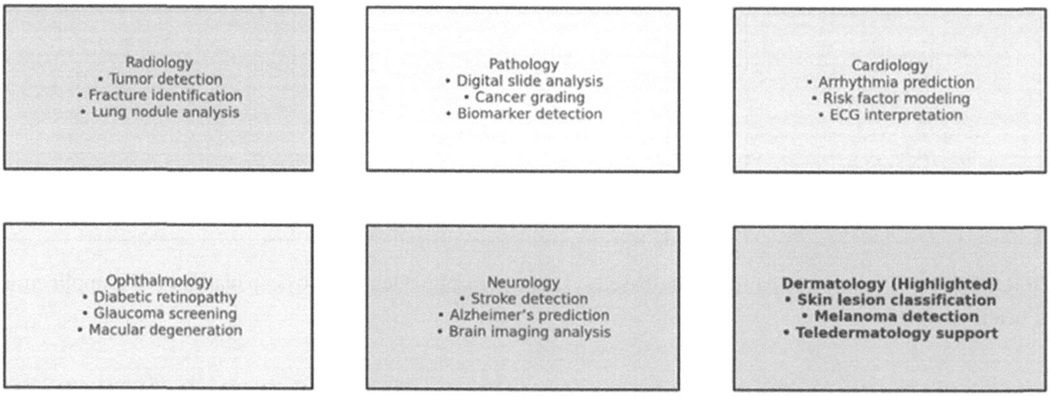

FIGURE 2.2 Applications of AI across healthcare specialties, highlighting dermatology.

morphologies. AI's strength in pattern recognition makes it a very valuable support in dermatology. For example:

- CNNs trained on the Human Against Machine with 10000 training images (HAM10000) or International Skin Imaging Collaboration (ISIC) archive datasets are on par with the best dermatologists in the field for melanoma detection.
- Teledermatology services utilize AI to carry out the initial screening of skin lesions, thus saving the specialists' time by directing only the most critical cases to them.
- AI-based mobile applications allow users to take pictures of their skin lesions using their smartphones and get instant evaluations of the risk of those lesions, making it possible, in a way, for early diagnosis to be performed even in underprivileged areas.

2.1.5 Ethical and Practical Considerations

The utilization of AI in dermatology is a topic that brings up some significant issues despite its advantages:

- Bias and fairness: Several AI systems are developed with a major reliance on photographs featuring fair-skinned persons, which results in inferior performance on darker skins.
- Interpretability: The black-box nature of the models creates a lack of trust among doctors. Currently, there is a growing interest in one of the Explainable AI (XAI) methods, which uses heat maps to show the areas in the lesions that the AI is focusing on during the decision-making.
- Regulation and integration: The introduction of an AI system into a clinical setting entails getting regulatory approval, ensuring compatibility with the hospital IT systems, training the medical staff, and so on.

AI has been developed over the years, moving through the stages of mathematical formulation to practical and clinical application. And among the different areas of medicine, AI has found rapid adoption in dermatology because of the visuality of skin disease diagnosis. The adoption of AI in healthcare has been limited by difficulties like biases, lack of transparent algorithms, and the need for regulatory approval, but still, the technology is seen as a means to better diagnostics, higher-quality treatments, and wider accessibility to services. The upcoming parts will focus on the implementation of AI in skin cancer detection considering the aspects of data acquisition, augmentation, tools, and challenges.

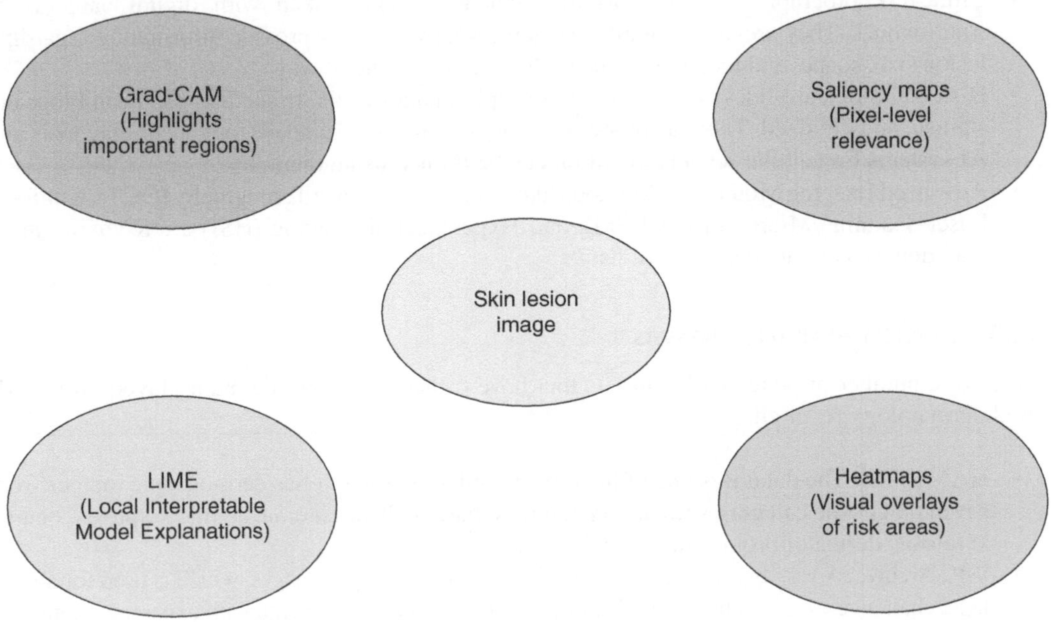

FIGURE 2.3 Role of explainable AI in skin cancer detection, showing heatmaps overlayed on lesion images.

2.2 DATA ACQUISITION

AI systems are primarily dependent on data and their performance is directly related to the quality, quantity, and diversity of the input data. In the area of dermatology and skin cancer detection, data collection is the main component of AI development. Where the traditional medical practice relies on the dermatologist's experience and intuition, AI systems need extensive training on carefully selected datasets to be able to detect patterns and give predictions.

2.2.1 Importance of Data in AI Systems

AI models, particularly the DL systems, need considerable amounts of annotated data so that they can perform accurately. In medical imaging, besides the image itself being able to show the relevant features, the image also needs to be provided with reliable labels. Usually, these labels are given by specialist dermatologists or through histopathology. In skin cancer detection, the dermoscopic images, clinical photographs, or histopathological slides usually make the datasets.

The presence of immense and accurately annotated datasets enables algorithms to be more reliable in different patient groups, lesion types, and imaging conditions. On the other hand, low-quality data or unbalanced datasets can result in biased predictions, which will in turn lower the utility of the solution and even bear risks.

2.2.2 Sources of Data

The imaging data of skin cancer can be taken from several sources:

- Dermoscopic Images: These images taken by handheld dermatoscopes show the subsurface structures of the skin which are not possible to see with the naked eye. Dermoscopy continues to be the most frequently used imaging technique for AI research in skin cancer.

- Clinical Photographs: It refers to the standard images taken with digital cameras or smartphones. They are not as detailed as dermoscopy, but they provide information regarding lesion size, shape, and location on the body in a more general way.
- Histopathological Slides: These are microscopic images of the tissue that has been biopsied, stained, and digitized. Their accuracy is considered the gold standard for cancer diagnosis and AI systems for cellular-level recognition can be trained using them.
- Advanced Imaging Modalities: Methods like Optical Coherence Tomography (OCT), Confocal Laser Scanning Microscopy (CLSM), and Hyperspectral Imaging (HSI) are receiving more attention as alternative sources of data.

2.2.3 Publicly Available Datasets

There are a number of benchmark datasets that have turned out to be the main players in the AI-based dermatology research:

- HAM10000: The dataset is one of the most popular ones and it has dermoscopic images from seven diagnostic categories (melanoma, nevus, basal cell carcinoma, actinic keratosis, benign keratosis, dermatofibroma, and vascular lesions).
- ISIC Archive: A very big open-access repository of dermoscopic images, which is used for annual ISIC challenges. It contains hundreds of thousands of images that come with expert annotations.
- PH2 Dataset: A smaller dataset with dermoscopic images, that is mainly focused on melanoma vs. benign nevi classification.
- Dermofit Image Library: It has more than 1,300 images covering 10 lesion classes that have been taken under standardized clinical conditions.

Algorithm comparison is one of the major uses of these datasets and they also play a very important role in the reproducibility of research.

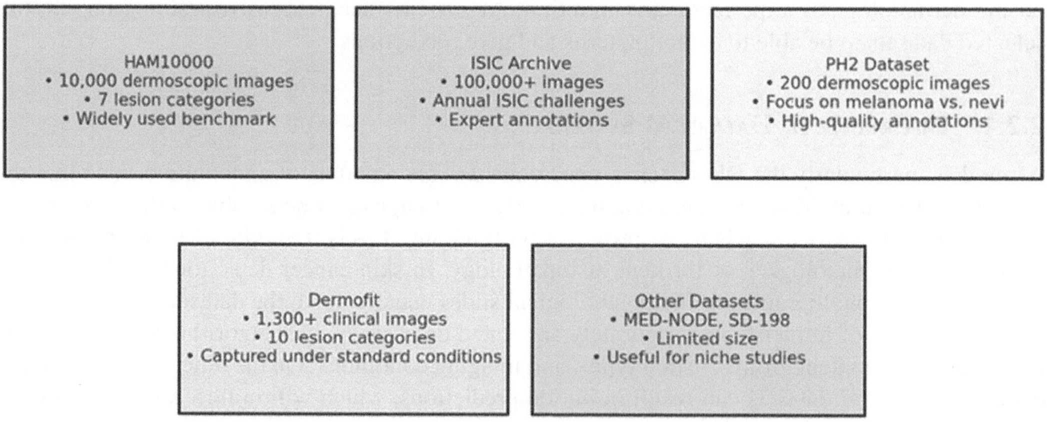

FIGURE 2.4 Examples of publicly available datasets used in skin cancer AI research (HAM10000, ISIC, PH2, Dermofit).

2.2.4 Challenges in Data Acquisition

Progress has been made, but there are still several challenges in the way of acquiring data suitable for AI systems:

- Data Imbalance: Certain lesion types (like melanoma) are much rarer than others (e.g., nevus). This situation causes the algorithms to predict common categories more than they should and, at the same time, to lose sensitivity towards rare but very important cancers.
- Diversity in the Population: The vast majority of the existing datasets have a bias towards fair-skinned persons, which makes the results from the data unapplicable to the population with darker skin tones. This, in turn, brings about ethical and clinical concerns about the whole issue of fairness and inclusivity.
- Annotation Accuracy: Labels are mainly derived from expert consensus or histopathology. The discrepancy among the dermatologists in terms of observing can contaminate the dataset with noise.
- Privacy and Ethics: Medical images are sensitive data. It is necessary to ensure patient anonymity and compliance with regulations like General Data Protection Regulation (GDPR) and Health Insurance Portability and Accountability Act (HIPAA) for responsible data usage.
- Data Standardization: The differences in imaging equipment, lighting, and resolution could lead to the creation of inconsistencies that will challenge the robustness of the algorithm.

2.2.5 Strategies for Improved Data Acquisition

Researchers tackle these problems using various approaches:

- Multi-Center Collaborations: Combining data from multiple hospitals and regions to improve the representativeness.
- Synthetic Data Generation: Using techniques like Generative Adversarial Networks (GANs) to create life-like synthetic dermoscopic images that balance out the underrepresented classes.
- Federated Learning: A privacy-preserving method where AI models are trained on disjoint datasets, and patient data is not disclosed in unprocessed form.
- Longitudinal Data Collection: Following up on the same patient across a timeline to record tumor modification and responsiveness to therapy.

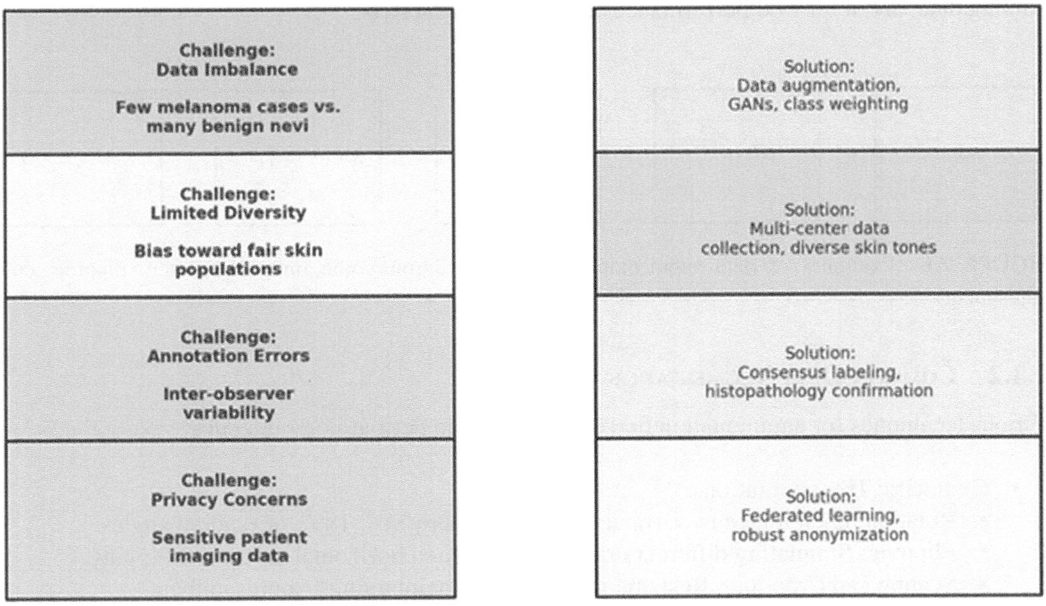

FIGURE 2.5 Challenges and solutions in data acquisition for skin cancer AI.

Data collection is the primary step to AI-based skin cancer detection. Quality, variety, and proper data annotation are the requirements for building models having good performance across different population groups and clinical environments. The situation is similar in case of public datasets such as HAM10000 and ISIC that have been very helpful in research but the problems of imbalance, diversity, and ethics still remain. New methods like federated learning and synthetic data generation are the ones that could overcome these challenges. In the end, the dermatologist's reliance on AI will not be just on superior algorithms but on the power of the data which is strong and representative enough to support those algorithms.

2.3 DATA AUGMENTATION AND PROCESSING

Data acquisition constitutes the primary unprocessed layer for the implementation of AI applications in dermatology; nevertheless, unprocessed medical images are hardly ever fit for the direct application in DL models. Their quality, resolution, orientation, and illumination frequently differ from each other. In addition, medical datasets are characteristically marked by the situation of class imbalance that is, malignant cases are not represented sufficiently in proportion to benign lesions. The aforementioned problems of data augmentation and preprocessing, which are the necessary steps to enhancing the robustness, generalization, and clinical applicability of AI models, have to be addressed first.

2.3.1 Importance of Data Augmentation

Data augmentation is an essential method of artificially increasing the size and diversity of a dataset by applying various transformations to the currently available images. In contrast to the traditional approach of collecting more raw data—which can be an expensive process and also subject to legal restrictions regarding privacy—augmentation provides a means to create variations that a model can encounter in real-life situations.

A dermoscopic image of a nevus, for instance, can be rotated, flipped, or color-adjusted to approximate the variations due to the change in patient posture, lighting, or imaging equipment. Consequently, augmentation leads to better generalization by the models, less sensitivity to specific training data, and improved performance across various datasets.

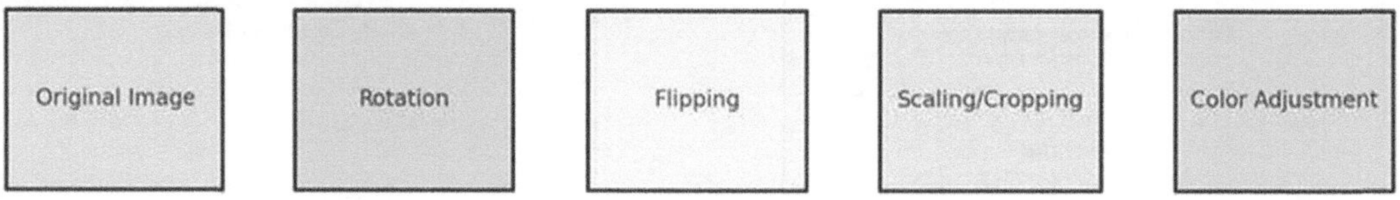

FIGURE 2.6 Examples of data augmentation applied to dermoscopic images (rotation, flipping, color adjustment).

2.3.2 Common Data Augmentation Techniques

Various techniques for augmentation find extensive use in dermatology imaging:

- Geometric Transformations:
  - Rotation: Each image is warranted to be rotated by 90°, 180°, or random angles.
  - Flipping: Simulating different orientations through horizontal or vertical flipping.
  - Scaling and Cropping: Resizing images while maintaining features in them.

- Photometric Adjustments:
  - Brightness and Contrast Variations: Simulating changes in lighting.
  - Color Jittering: Randomly changing hue, saturation, or intensity.
- Noise Injection:
  - Gaussian or salt-and-pepper noise added to the image thus simulating real-world image imperfections.
- Elastic Transformations:
  - Slightly warping or distorting the images to mimic biological variability in lesions.
- Synthetic Image Generation:
  - GANs and other advanced techniques make it possible to create realistic synthetic skin lesion images, hence, aiding the rare classes like melanoma which need augmentation.

2.3.3 Preprocessing for Skin Cancer Images

Preprocessing, among other things, made output images ready for efficient training of the model:

- Image Normalization: Making all the pixel values within a fixed range (for instance, 0–1) to avoid issues with numerical instability.
- Resizing: Making all the input dimensions uniform (e.g., 224×224 for ResNet).
- Color Normalization: Making sure that the colors of the images taken by different devices are the same.
- Hair Removal: Algorithms (e.g., DullRazor) are used to get rid of hair artifacts that might hide lesion boundaries.
- Segmentation: Employing thresholding, clustering (k-means), and DL architectures (U-Net, Mask R-CNN) for the identification of lesion boundaries. Segmentation technique separates the lesion from adjacent skin which in turn increases the accuracy of classification.

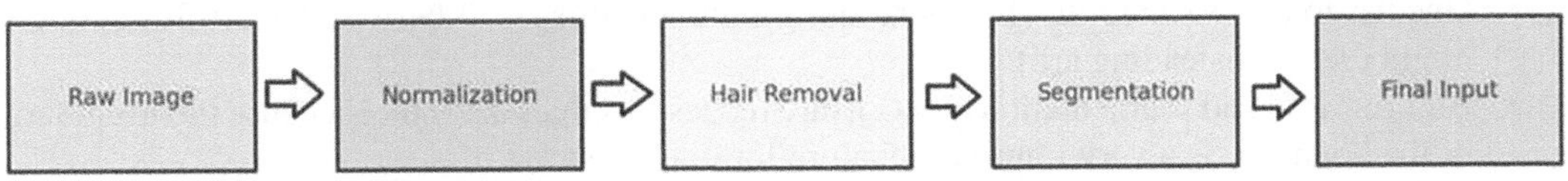

FIGURE 2.7 Preprocessing workflow: raw image → normalization → hair removal → segmentation → final input.

2.3.4 Data Balancing Strategies

Tumors that are not benign (like melanoma, for example) are quite rare in clinical practice and datasets, so it is very important to balance:

- Minority Classes Oversampling: Making copies or augmenting images of rare classes.
- Majority Classes Undersampling: Reducing the number of benign lesions which are common.
- Class Weights: During model training, minority classes are given higher weights for misclassification.
- Synthetic Oversampling (SMOTE): New synthetic examples are generated by interpolating between the existing samples.

The use of different strategies for balancing the data keeps the models from being biased towards the categories that are represented the most.

2.3.5 Processing Pipeline for AI Systems

In real-world situations, data augmentation and preprocessing are the main steps of a pipeline that carries out the following activities:

1. Raw Image Collection (clinical/dermoscopic/histopathology).
2. Preprocessing (resizing, normalization, hair removal).
3. Segmentation (optional, isolates lesion).
4. Augmentation (rotations, flips, synthetic images).
5. Final Dataset Preparation (balanced, high-quality images ready for training).

This systematic process guarantees conformity, productivity, and reproducibility among studies.

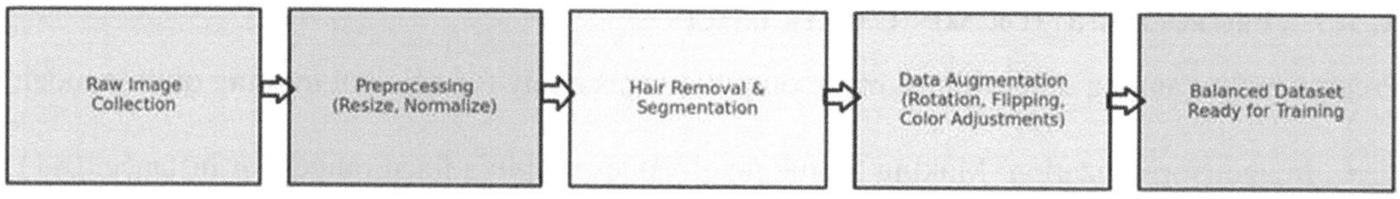

FIGURE 2.8 Workflow diagram of data processing and augmentation for skin cancer AI.

2.3.6 Clinical Considerations in Augmentation and Processing

On the one hand, augmentation boosts technical performance, but on the other hand, the clinical context is still very important:

- Overly aggressive transformations can change the shape of the tumor, and thus, provide samples that are not realistic biologically.
- One has to be very careful while generating synthetic images; otherwise the artificial patterns might create misleading artifacts.
- Hair removal and segmentation must ensure the lesion edges are intact because the irregularity of the boundary is a very important feature for diagnosis.

Properly conceived augmentation and preprocessing methods not only improve AI models but also keep them in line with clinical practice.

In the process of AI-supported skin cancer diagnosis, data augmentation and preprocessing are critical steps. The first of these techniques, for instance, enhances the quality of the model in terms of accuracy and reliability by increasing the diversity of the dataset, fixing the image artifacts, and making sure that each class is well-represented. Among the methods used for data augmentation are simple geometric transformations and complex GAN-based synthesis, which all work together with data acquisition to overcome the challenges that medical datasets impose. These two processes together ensure that the establishment of AI solutions in dermatology that are powerful, scalable, and clinically applicable is not too difficult.

2.4 AI TOOLS AND REQUIREMENTS

The successful application of AI for skin cancer detection relies not just on data of high quality and algorithms that work effectively, but also on the development-supporting tools, frameworks, and infrastructure. In this part, the critical AI instruments, programming settings, hardware demands, and workflows are mentioned that allow both researchers and clinicians to construct as well as assess strong AI systems for dermatology.

2.4.1 AI Development Frameworks

Over the last ten years, the emergence of open-source tools has changed the landscape of AI research completely. The innovation process has been speeded up and at the same time, the cost of entering the field has been drastically reduced. The principal open-source frameworks are:

- TensorFlow (Google): A large-scale ML platform that is flexible and powerful, supporting not only DL but also dataflow graphs and distributed training. The integration of Keras offers a user-friendly API.
- PyTorch (Meta AI): A dynamic, Pythonic framework that spots the advantage of easy-going experimentation. It has turned into the researchers' tool of choice in the academic field and is also catching the favor of the industry.
- Keras: An easy-to-use high-level API that makes the creation of DL models easier and often is used together with TensorFlow.
- Scikit-learn: A classical ML library that presents algorithms for classification, regression, clustering, and preprocessing and is predominantly used in feature-based models.
- MXNet and CNTK: Rarely used today, but they have been praised for their capabilities in scalability and support for distributed computing.

Now, in the area of AI in dermatology, TensorFlow and PyTorch have monopolized the market as they provide excellent support for CNNs, transfer learning, and the use of pre-trained models.

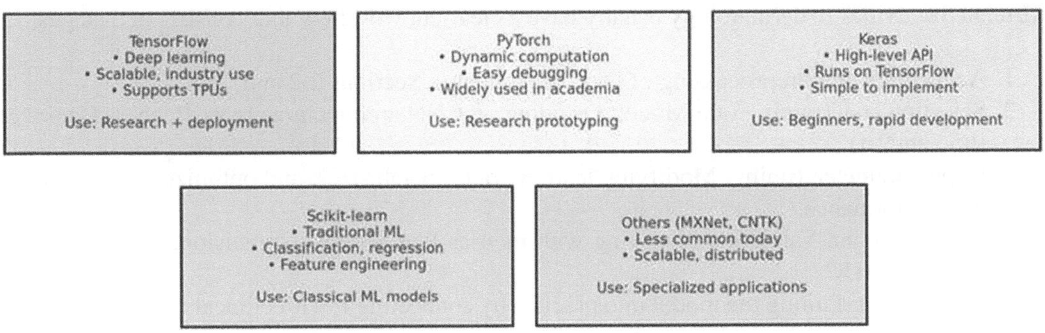

FIGURE 2.9 Comparison of AI frameworks (TensorFlow, PyTorch, Keras, Scikit-learn) and their use cases.

2.4.2 Hardware Requirements

The application of DL methods, specifically CNNs, means the consumption of considerable system resources. The major hardware issues are as follows:

- CPUs (Central Processing Units): This type of unit is good when it comes to small experiments and conventional ML models, yet it is commonly not enough for training deep CNNs.
- GPUs (Graphics Processing Units): These are designed specifically for doing parallel computations and thus, GPUs effectively lead to a remarkable reduction in time to perform DL; NVIDIA's CUDA-enabled GPUs are the preferred hardware in AI research.

- TPUs (Tensor Processing Units): Google has come up with TPUs which are tailored to TensorFlow workloads and thus, they are super efficient when it comes to providing cloud-based training.
- Memory and Storage: Huge datasets like ISIC archive can cause the storage needed to be in the range of terabytes. The data loading times are cut down by using fast SSDs. The training of large CNNs needs GPUs having at least 8–16 GB of VRAM.
- Cloud Platforms: Google Cloud, AWS, Microsoft Azure, and other similar services offer the advantages of having a scalable set up with the availability of the GPUs and TPUs for the researchers to train models without incurring the cost of very costly local hardware.

2.4.3 Software and Programming Environments

- Python: The main programming language for AI researches, thus got support through wide-ranging libraries for data science (NumPy, Pandas, Matplotlib).
- Jupyter Notebooks: The interactive coding environments that are perfect for prototyping and visualization.
- Docker and Virtual Environments: Ensured reproducibility and portability of AI workflows as part of the toolset.

To give an idea of the tools and their usability in AI research, the mentioned aspects will be considered first and then the availability of the research area to non-computer-scientists such as clinicians will be highlighted.

2.4.4 Workflow of AI Model Development

AI-related activities in dermatology usually have a clear-cut workflow that consists of 5 stages:

1. Acquisition and Preprocessing of Data (treatment in Sections 2.2 and 2.3).
2. Selection and Training of a Model: Deciding on CNN architectures (e.g., ResNet, DenseNet, EfficientNet).
3. Hyperparameter Tuning: Modifying learning rates, batch sizes, and optimizer settings for the best performance.
4. Evaluation and Validation: Tracking with metrics like accuracy, precision, recall, F1-score, and ROC-AUC.
5. Deployment: Putting the model into practice by connecting it with clinical systems or making it available through mobile app usage.

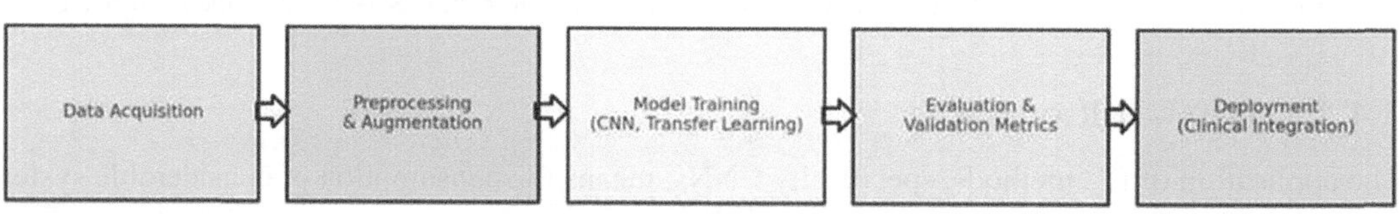

FIGURE 2.10 Workflow of AI development for skin cancer detection: data → preprocessing → training → evaluation → deployment.

2.4.5 Transfer Learning and Pretrained Models

The process of training DL models from the start is quite demanding in terms of computational power, and it is not always necessary. Researchers, instead, employ transfer learning, which means that the models already trained on large datasets (like ImageNet) are adjusted to work better on smaller medical datasets, such as HAM10000 or ISIC.

- Advantages:
  - It significantly reduces both training time and hardware expenditures.
  - It gives a performance boost in the scenario of inadequate labeled medical data.
- Popular Architectures: ResNet, VGG, Inception, DenseNet, EfficientNet.

Transfer learning has been the prevailing method in medical imaging AI. As a consequence, the creation of high-performance models that are easier to obtain has been accelerated.

2.4.6 Clinical Integration Requirements

Before AI systems could be applied in clinical practice, they had to pass a few more requirements:

- Interoperability: Integration of AI tools with hospital-related information systems (HIS) and EHRs is a must.
- User Interface Design: Creation of clinician-friendly dashboards that show predictions with explanations (e.g., heatmaps) is more than necessary.
- Regulatory Approval: Meeting the standards of FDA (USA), CE marking (Europe), and CDSCO (India) is a must.
- Security and Privacy: To ensure patient data protection, compliance with HIPAA and GDPR needs to be guaranteed.

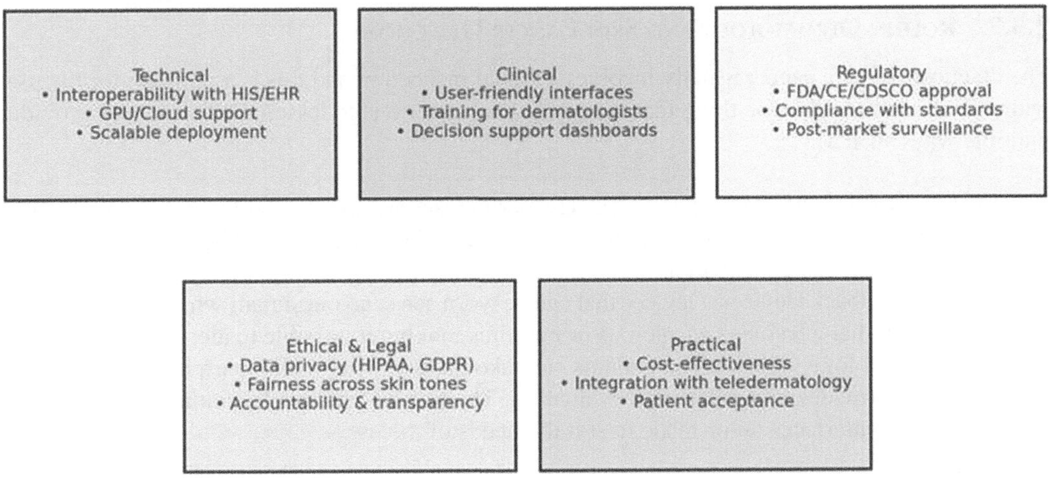

FIGURE 2.11 Requirements for integrating AI into dermatology practice (technical, regulatory, clinical, ethical).

AI tools along with their requisite infrastructure do not only imply the use of algorithms but also the framework, hardware, software, and integration pipelines. TensorFlow and PyTorch have remained the main research frameworks, whereas GPUs and cloud services have been the main providers of the necessary computational power. Transfer learning is the technique that links the small medical datasets with the need for very precise models. Moreover, for the clinicians to trust the AI systems, interoperability, interpretability, and regulatory approval are all musts. This amalgamation of technology and clinical demands guarantees that AIs are integrated into dermatology with the utmost reliability, thus making it possible for the technology to have a real impact on the market.

2.5 USE OF AI FOR IMPAIRED USERS ASSISTANCE

AI is transforming not only diagnostics and planning of treatments but also becoming a major factor in assistive technologies for the disabled. These technological advances allow accessibility to healthcare and empower the healthcare staff and patients who are limited by visual, auditory, or motor disabilities. In the field of dermatology, the tools for detecting skin cancer based on AI can be redesigned for use by both the doctors who have disabilities and the patients who need inclusive medical support.

2.5.1 AI in Assistive Healthcare

The potential of AI-assisted support systems is enormous not only in skin cancer diagnosis but also in other areas of healthcare:

- The use of AI-supported computer vision enables blind users to identify objects, read texts, and receive descriptions of scenes through smartphones or wearables.
- The hearing impaired are benefiting from NLP technology through real-time captioning and sign language interpreting.
- In the case of the physically handicapped, AI voice assistants are doing hands-free operations for medical devices and patient monitoring tools.

These cases illustrate the great contribution of AI in making healthcare accessible to all and in establishing a fair healthcare system.

2.5.2 Role in Dermatology and Skin Cancer Detection

The diagnosis of skin cancer usually involves a visual inspection and this is a problem for the users with visual impairment. One thing that the AI systems can do is to lessen the barriers by providing multiple ways such as:

- Voice-Assisted Diagnostic Feedback: The dermatoscopic apps that are integrated with AI can describe aloud the risk of the lesion (for instance, "The lesion is likely benign" or "High risk, seek dermatology consultation").
- Haptic Feedback Devices: Devices that can be worn can send out signals which can be felt indicating whether a lesion is suspicious or not, thus making it possible to alert non-visual ways.
- Teledermatology with AI: The patients can take pictures with their smartphones while the AI software provides immediate risk evaluation. The results can then be communicated through accessible interfaces tailor-made to suit the needs of the users.

2.5.3 AI for Clinicians with Impairments

In addition, AI is capable of assisting healthcare professionals who are impaired, thus allowing them to keep on practicing successfully:

- Motor-impaired radiologists might depend on the AI systems for automatic image segmentation.
- AI maps and probability scores intended for the visually impaired can be used as additional tools in the doctor's evaluation for dermatologists with partial sight.
- Decision-support dashboards give easy-to-read and simplified summaries of AI predictions, thus minimizing cognitive and sensory load.

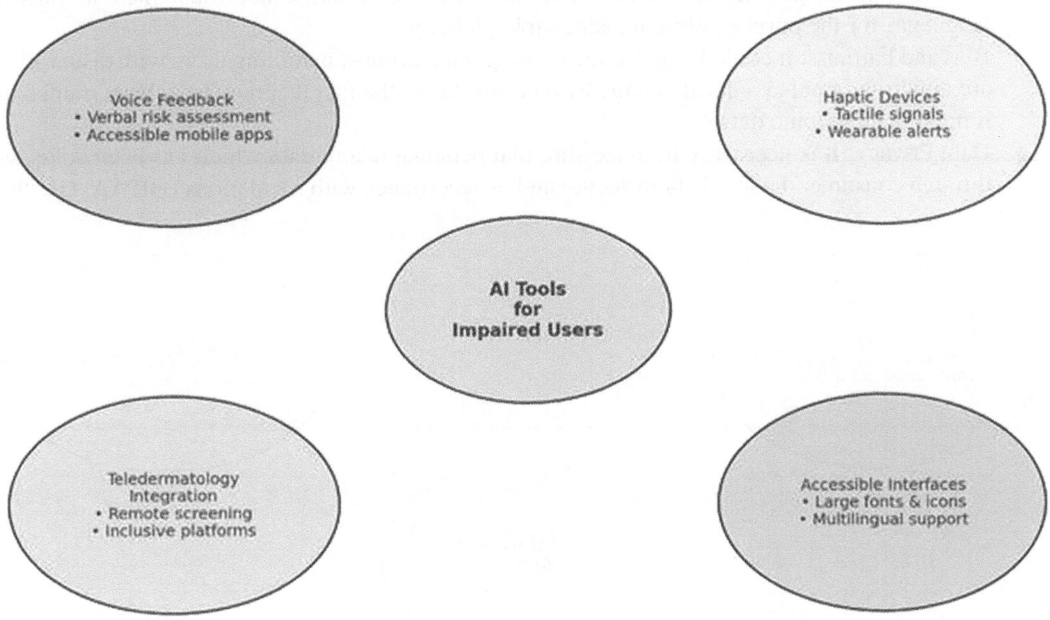

FIGURE 2.12 AI-assisted tools for impaired users: voice feedback, haptic devices, teledermatology integration.

By cutting down reliance on visual-only reading, AI opens up the medical workforce to people with different abilities.

2.5.4 Integration with Consumer Devices

The consumer electronics industry is very important for the application of AI-based assistance to disabled users:

- Smartphones: They have high-quality cameras and features that help users with disabilities (like voice assistants, screen readers).
- Smart Glasses and Wearables: OrCam and Microsoft Seeing AI are already capable of recognizing objects; it is possible to apply the same technology to skin lesion analysis.
- Home Assistants: Through the collaboration with Alexa or Google Assistant, it would be possible to create a voice-based system for lesion monitoring and scheduling of appointments.

These integrations not only support the trend of patient-centered healthcare but also give power to the patients to take full control over their health.

2.5.5 Ethical and Social Considerations

In spite of the fact that AI comes with the promise of inclusivity, its usage still has to deal with ethical and social issues:

- Accessibility Equity: The systems must be cost-effective and flexible enough to accommodate users from all financial backgrounds.

- Cultural and Linguistic Adaptation: The output of voice assistance must include various languages for the purpose of being accessible globally.
- Bias and Fairness: It could be that some demographic groups, including users with disabilities, are unwittingly put at a disadvantage by AI tools due to the fact that they have been trained on limited demographic data.
- Data Privacy: It is necessary to make sure that personal health data which has been collected through consumer devices is both secure and in accordance with regulations (HIPAA, GDPR).

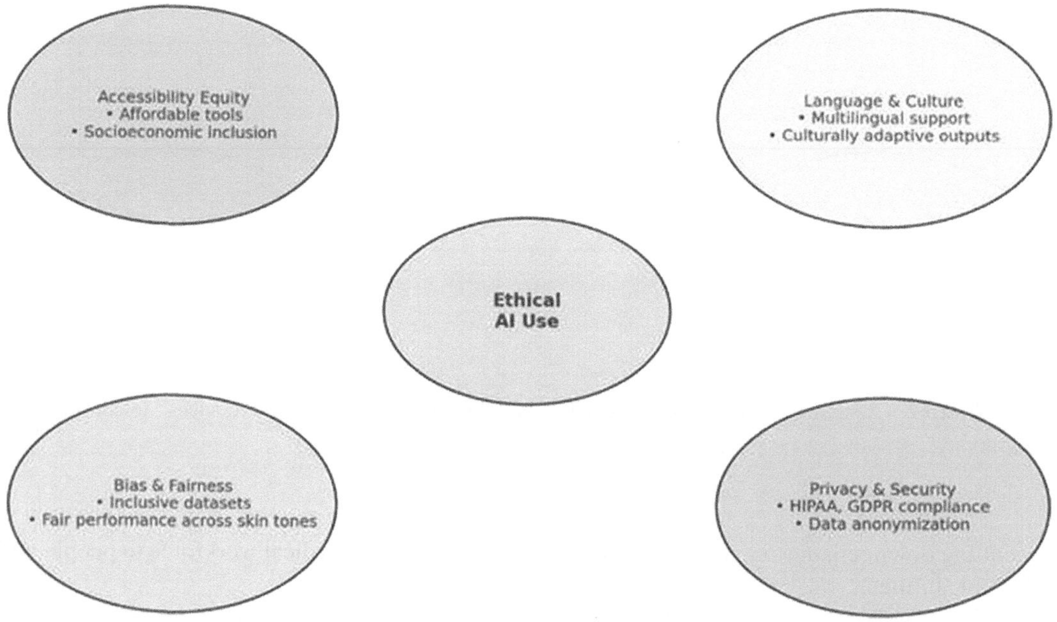

FIGURE 2.13 Ethical considerations in AI for impaired users (equity, language, bias, privacy).

2.5.6 Case Studies and Emerging Applications

- Be My Eyes (AI Integration): A mobile application that pairs users with visual impairments with volunteers who can see, has now incorporated AI to offer immediate help.
- Skin Cancer AI Apps with Voice Feedback: The prototypes from the study give the risk level of the lesion orally, hence, making the self-examination process easier.
- Wearable AI for Continuous Monitoring: The trial gadgets keep track of the skin condition over a certain period and notify the users about the formation or alteration of the lesions.

These examples of AI in dermatology and other areas emphasize the practicality of the technology for disabled users.

The application of AI to people with disabilities marks a very important move to inclusive healthcare. By making the diagnostic tools suitable for the different kinds of users with the help of voice output, tactile feedback, and consumer device integration, AI lets patients and doctors having the same impairments reap the benefits of dermatology improvements. Among such innovations, ethical aspects like these—affordability, fairness, and privacy—should be the pioneers in order not to drive new inequities. In the end, AI may not only be the main factor in improving skin cancer detection but also in providing healthcare access to the disabled all around the globe.

2.6 ISSUES AND CHALLENGES

On the one hand, the dermatology field and skin cancer identification have gained a lot from AI or Artificial Intelligence; on the other hand, its use in clinical practice encounters numerous problems. The obstacles are of technical, clinical, ethical, and regulatory nature. It is important to overcome them in order to make AI tools reach that high degree of precision not only in research control but also in healthcare systems worldwide, being therefore safe, trustworthy, and fair.

2.6.1 Data-Related Challenges

The performance of AI systems heavily depends on the quality of their training data. In the field of dermatology, data-related problems are still the main obstacles:

- Dataset Imbalance: In real-world datasets, malignant lesions like melanoma are much scarcer than benign nevi. This long-standing problem causes model predictions to be completely misdirected, with the result that poor sensitivity is often the case for rare but vital cancers.
- Limited Diversity: Datasets that are publicly accessible (e.g., HAM10000, ISIC) mainly consist of images representing individuals with light skin. As a result, AI systems that are trained using these datasets might not provide accurate results when used on people with darker skin; thus, causing inequities in diagnosis.
- Annotation Quality: The assignment of labels is dependent on either the expertise of a dermatologist or histopathological verification. The inconsistency between different dermatologists can cause inaccurate labeling that will consequently be passed on to the AI models.
- Small Sample Sizes for Rare Lesions: There are a few categories of lesions (e.g., dermatofibroma, vascular lesions) that are seldom represented, and this makes it hard for AI to pick up the features that differentiate them.

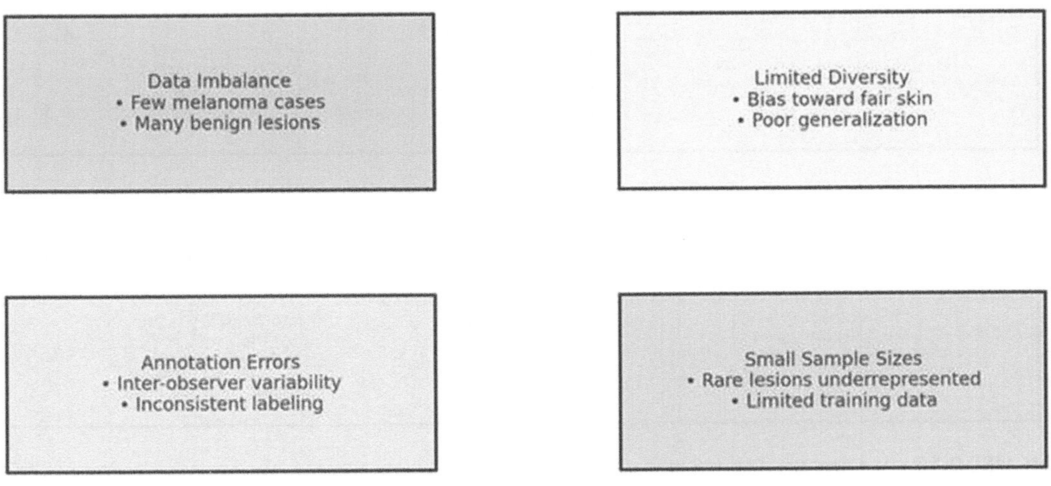

FIGURE 2.14 Data-related challenges in AI: imbalance, diversity, annotation quality.

2.6.2 Algorithmic Challenges

Even though high-quality data is available, algorithms are still facing the following challenges that are inherent in them:

- Overfitting: In the case of small datasets, DL models may learn the training data by heart rather than being able to generalize properly.
- Interpretability: A large number of AI systems behave like "black boxes" and give out predictions without giving any reason. The inability to interpret the results makes the clinicians lose trust, which in turn slows down the adoption process.
- Generalizability: A model that has been trained using one dataset might not work efficiently while processing images that come from different hospitals or using different devices or patient groups.
- Computational Demands: The computation power required for large CNNs is significant, and it might not be available in every clinical setting, especially the ones located in low-resource areas.

2.6.3 Clinical Integration Challenges

It is a complicated process to bring AI systems to the daily dermatology practice:

- Disruption of the Workflow: The AI tools have to be integrated in such a way that they do not disrupt the clinic's workflow and that they do not add too much complexity or time-consuming activities.
- Training of Users: Physicians need to be trained on how to read AI outputs, above all probabilities and heat maps.
- Patient Trust: Patients might be reluctant to accept AI-based diagnoses unless a doctor confirms them, thus requiring a combination of human and AI involvement.
- Interoperability: The AI tools have to be compatible with the current hospital information systems and electronic medical records.

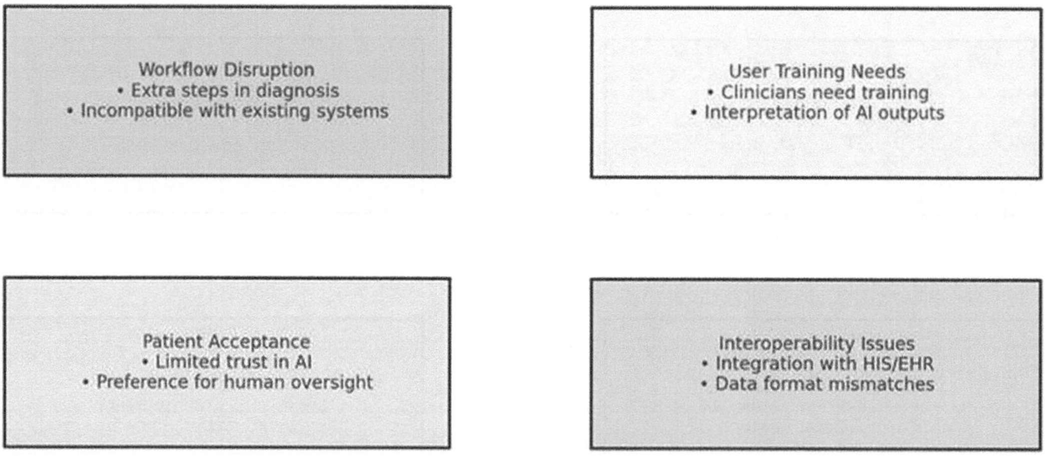

FIGURE 2.15 Barriers to AI adoption in clinical workflows.

2.6.4 Ethical and Legal Concerns

AI adoption raises important ethical and legal issues:

- **Bias and Fairness:** Models trained on biased datasets may inadvertently disadvantage minority populations. Ensuring fairness requires dataset diversification and algorithmic auditing.

- **Accountability:** In case of diagnostic errors, responsibility must be clearly defined—whether it lies with the clinician, the AI developer, or the institution.
- **Privacy:** Medical imaging involves sensitive patient data. Robust anonymization and compliance with privacy regulations (e.g., GDPR, HIPAA) are mandatory.
- **Transparency:** Patients and clinicians must be informed when AI is used as part of the diagnostic process, ensuring ethical transparency.

2.6.5 Regulatory and Policy Challenges

AI tools in dermatology must navigate a rigorous regulatory landscape:

- **FDA (United States):** The Food and Drug Administration regulates AI-based medical devices. Approval requires demonstrating safety, efficacy, and clinical validity.
- **CE Marking (Europe):** European Union standards mandate compliance with medical device regulations before deployment.
- **CDSCO (India):** The Central Drugs Standard Control Organization governs medical software and device approvals in India.
- **Dynamic Nature of AI:** Unlike static medical devices, AI models can evolve as they learn from new data, raising questions about how to regulate continuously adapting systems.

2.6.6 Future Challenges and Opportunities

Addressing current challenges opens new opportunities for innovation:

- **XAI:** Techniques like Grad-CAM and saliency maps can highlight the regions of an image that influenced a prediction, improving transparency.
- **Federated Learning:** Training models across decentralized datasets without sharing raw data enhances privacy while improving diversity.
- **Edge AI:** Running lightweight models on smartphones and dermatoscopes can expand access in low-resource regions.
- **Ethical AI Frameworks:** Institutions are increasingly adopting frameworks for fairness, accountability, and transparency to guide responsible AI deployment.

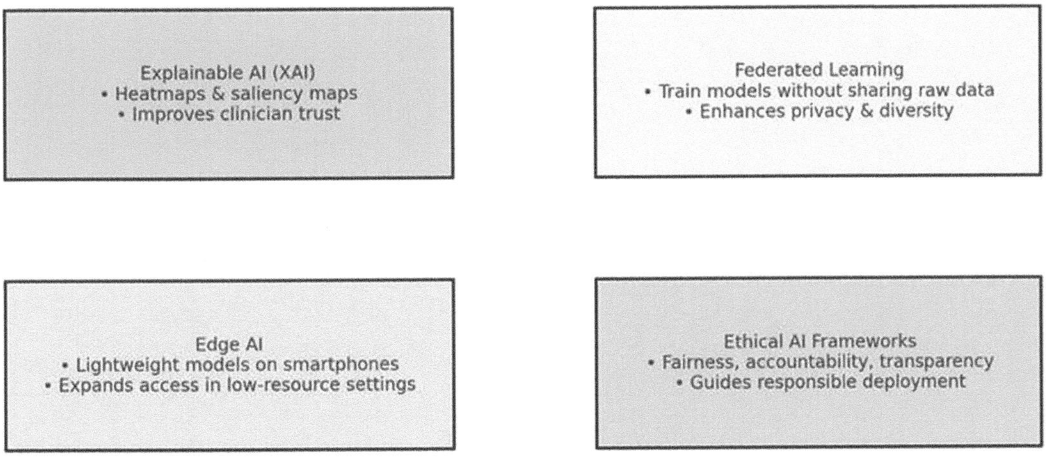

FIGURE 2.16 Opportunities for overcoming AI challenges: XAI, federated learning, edge AI.

The integration of AI into skin cancer detection faces a complex set of issues spanning data, algorithms, clinical practice, ethics, and regulation. Imbalanced and biased datasets, interpretability problems, workflow disruption, and unclear accountability remain key barriers. Yet, these challenges also provide opportunities for innovation, such as XAI, federated learning, and edge computing. For AI to achieve its full potential in dermatology, researchers, clinicians, policymakers, and technologists must collaborate to address these issues holistically. Only then can AI systems evolve from promising prototypes to trusted clinical partners in the fight against skin cancer.

3 AI for Skin Cancer Identification

3.1 PUBLIC HEALTH SAFETY USING ARTIFICIAL INTELLIGENCE

Skin cancer is a rapidly increasing global health burden, with its incidence overtaking that of most other cancers. In this sense, artificial intelligence (AI) is not just a diagnostic revolution but also a public health protector that can change early detection, risk evaluation, and access to healthcare.

3.1.1 AI AS A PUBLIC HEALTH ENABLER

AI facilitates dermatology care decentralization by running screening programs at the community level. The major techniques for detection, visual examination, and biopsy, are quite costly and require a high level of skill from dermatologists, who are usually available in urban areas. With the use of AI-powered screening tools, the healthcare system can go as far as rural and underserved communities, where early detection is most difficult.

AI algorithms that have been trained on thousands of dermoscopic images can recognize and categorize lesions as either malignant or benign. If these models are used in telemedicine settings, then they can lead to a three-tier public health strategy:

1. Awareness and Prevention – Mobile applications that use AI help to protect users from UV radiation by tracking their exposure and reminding them of protection measures.
2. Screening and Detection – Community health workers or people take pictures of the lesions for AI-based triage that is automated.
3. Clinical Referral and Monitoring – Only those cases that are of high risk are sent to dermatologists for further assessment and biopsy.

This method, which is capable of being widely applied, could ameliorate a lot the problem of diagnostic delays, which are very important for melanoma prognosis.

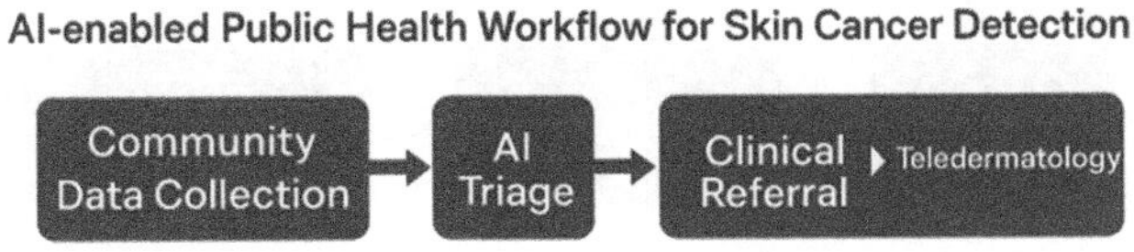

FIGURE 3.1 AI-enabled public health workflow for skin cancer detection integrating community data collection, AI triage, and teledermatology.

DOI: 10.1201/9781003542155-3

3.1.2 Epidemiological Surveillance with AI

AI techniques can analyze and combine non-personalized diagnostic data to keep an eye on disease incidence patterns in different areas. When combined with geospatial data, predictive analytics can create a map showing UV intensity, at-risk people, and changing skin cancer occurrences. These insights can be utilized by the government and health authorities for directing their prevention efforts and distributing their resources.

3.1.3 Ethical and Regulatory Considerations

Though the advantages are enormous, AI-based public health measures will have to face the following crucial issues:

- Data Protection – Patient photographs and their details have to be in line with the regulations of GDPR and HIPAA.
- Algorithmic Prejudice – A large number of AI applications give less than satisfactory results for patients with dark skin because the datasets are unbalanced.
- Opacity – Doctors need to be acquainted with the reasoning behind the model in order to be sure of the accountability.

In order to promote ethical integration, guidelines which are based on XAI and Federated Learning are recommended. These make it possible to train models locally without having to transfer patients' data, thus increasing both privacy and fairness.

3.2 SAFETY PRECAUTIONS FOR SKIN CANCER

A complete procedure for skin cancer prevention that is behaviorally educational, environmentally protective, and AI-assisted self-monitoring is used. Preventive care's collaboration with AI is the core of an advanced medical public health model.

3.2.1 Lifestyle and Environmental Precautions

UV radiation exposure is still the foremost risk factor for skin cancer. Applications for smartphones using AI now act as digital partners in prevention. Through integrating UV-index forecasts, AI models can do the following:

- Provide alerts in real-time to reduce sun exposure,
- Suggest intervals for sunscreen application,
- Use computer vision to identify skin color for personalized recommendations, and
- Monitor over time to spot early suspicious changes in existing moles.

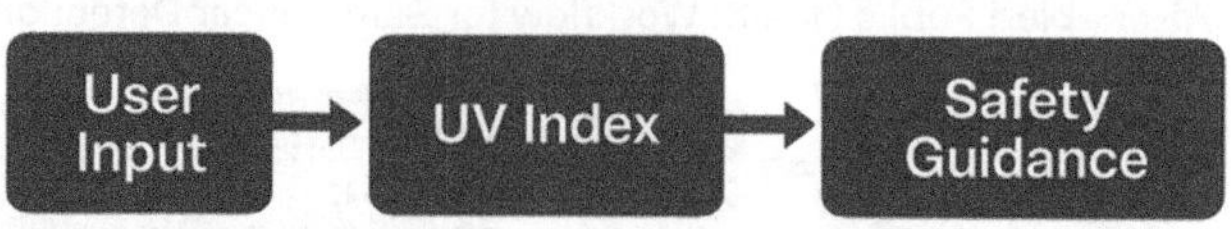

FIGURE 3.2 AI-based UV risk assessment and lifestyle recommendation system for individual safety.

These applications combine **computer vision**, **geolocation**, and **reinforcement learning** to provide personalized and adaptive preventive care.

3.2.2 AI in Occupational Health and Risk Prediction

Workers in the construction, agriculture, or outdoor industries are continuously exposed to UV rays. Wearable IoT sensors combined with AI algorithms will be able to provide the continuous measurement of the total UV dose, skin temperature, and the level of environmental intensity. Time-series analysis together with predictive models can be used to send alerts in case of high-risk exposure patterns. In big companies, AI-powered risk dashboards summarize the data on employee exposure to guarantee adherence to the occupational safety regulations, which is a way of preventing the dangerous effects of cancer over a long period of time.

3.2.3 Skin Self-Examination and AI Assistance

Skin self-examinations are widely regarded as an inevitable preventive measure by the American Cancer Society and WHO. AI-powered smartphone cameras that come with lesion monitoring algorithms can analyze specifics like shape, color, asymmetry, and border irregularity constantly and give an automated ABCDE evaluation (Asymmetry, Border, Color, Diameter, Evolution) of the lesion's status.

Thus, this dispersal of diagnostic intelligence has a positive effect on early detection through self-exams, thus decreasing the number of patients who come in the later stages of the disease.

3.3 AI MODEL BUILDING FOR SKIN CANCER DETECTION

To build a powerful AI model capable of detecting skin cancers, it is necessary to rely upon a solid and evidence-based strategy that utilizes clinical imaging, data science, and ML. This part of the text combines not only the general AI method but also the specific experimental contributions of Ingle (2023), PhD Thesis, SPPU.

3.3.1 Dataset and Preprocessing

The model efficiently combines datasets that consist of HAM10000, PH2, and the dermoscopic images that were collected in the clinical setting through controlled trials. After going through the processes of augmentation, normalization, and noise correction, 25,000 images were ready for use in total.

The main preprocessing operations included:

- Changing the size of the images to 224×224 pixels.
- Applying histogram equalization for color normalization aimed at equalizing luminance and contrast.
- Cutting out hair artifacts by using DullRazor followed by morphological filtering.
- Using a Modified SegNet architecture for segmentation to separate lesions from the surrounding skin—boundary detection.
- The SegNet produced an IoU of 0.93 and a Dice Coefficient of 0.95 thereby surpassing the performance of traditional thresholding and k-means methods, and consequently improving the accuracy of the subsequent classification.

The proposed research framework aspires to construct an automated skin cancer detection system from medical images employing AI through an integrated three-phase approach: segmentation, classification, and explainability. The first step concerns the adoption of SegNet, a deep convolutional

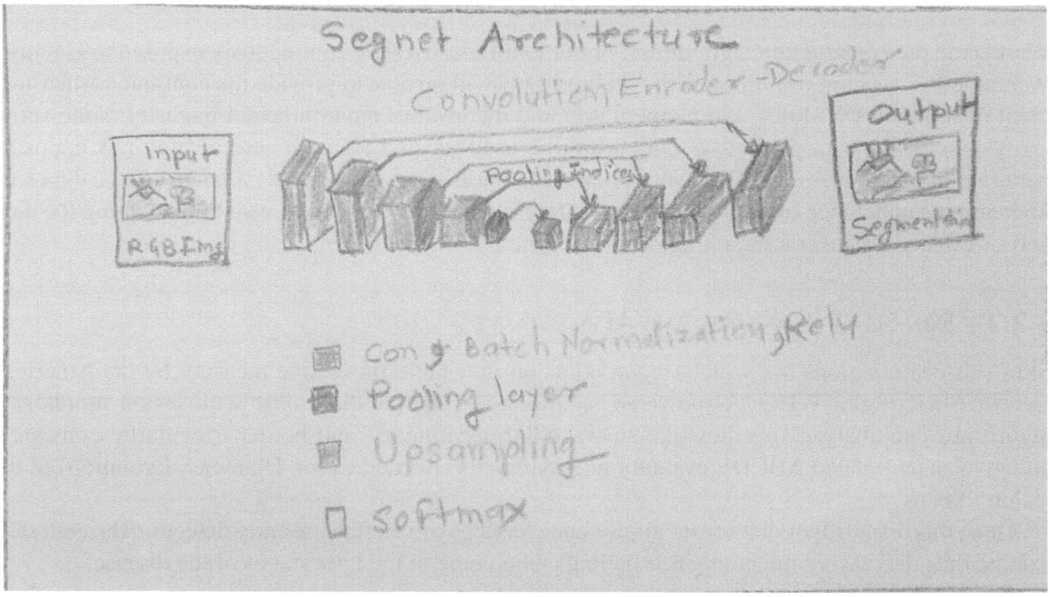

FIGURE 3.3 SegNet-based segmentation output demonstrating clear lesion.

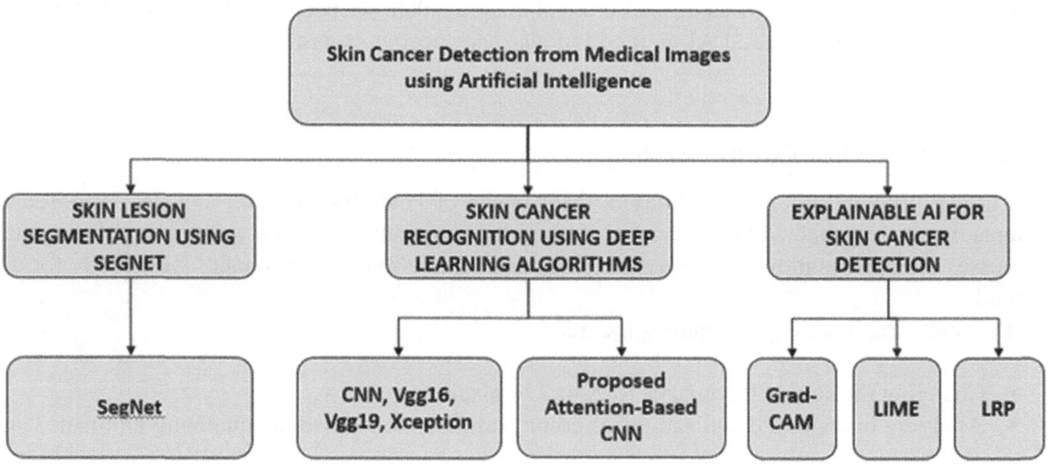

FIGURE 3.4 Research outline.

encoder-decoder network, for skin lesion segmentation, which eliminates the surrounding skin and gives the lesion area a clearer view for better precision of further analysis. The segmentation is so accurate that it enables the model to concentrate on the most important diagnostic features, thus, improving the performance of the classification done afterwards.

The second step concentrates on skin cancer detection using sophisticated deep learning architectures. Different CNN-based models like VGG16, VGG19, and Xception are analyzed for their capability to extract features and their classification accuracies. An Attention-Based Convolutional Neural Network (ABCNN) is proposed grounded on this to direct the spatial focus on the malignant regions by combining an attention mechanism. The third phase brings in XAI methods—Grad-CAM, LIME, and Layer-wise Relevance Propagation (LRP)—to make the results comprehensible visually and provide assurance of clinical honesty. The modules collectively develop a robust, explainable, and scalable framework that has the capability of achieving high diagnostic accuracy while at the same time, trust and accountability are being maintained in AI-assisted dermatological systems.

3.3.2 Model Architectures Evaluated

Multiple deep learning models were evaluated for lesion classification:

TABLE 3.1
Performance Comparison of Evaluated Deep Learning Architectures

Model	Parameters	Accuracy (%)	F1-Score	Inference Time (ms)
CNN (Baseline)	3.5 M	89.2	0.87	65
VGG16	138 M	91.7	0.90	92
VGG19	143 M	92.4	0.91	88
Xception	23 M	94.1	0.93	74
Proposed ABCNN	18 M	**98.6**	**0.98**	**70**

The **ABCNN** demonstrated superior performance owing to its *spatial attention layer*, which dynamically focused on diagnostically relevant regions, and a *residual skip connection* that preserved contextual information.

Mathematically, attention weight α_i was computed as:

$$\alpha_i = \frac{e^{W_i^T h_i}}{\sum_j e^{W_j^T h_j}}$$

where W_i denotes learnable attention parameters and h_i the feature map activations.

3.3.3 Explainable Artificial Intelligence (XAI) Framework

For the sake of model understanding and trust in the medical field, different XAI methods were combined, namely:

- Grad-CAM for visualizing the most important areas,
- LIME for determining which features are responsible for the prediction, and
- LRP for support of the heatmap produced.

These explainability layers allow dermatologists to verify model logic and identify misclassification trends, aligning with ethical AI principles.

3.3.4 Evaluation Metrics and Validation

Performance was assessed through **10-fold cross-validation** and evaluated on unseen test data. The following metrics were considered:

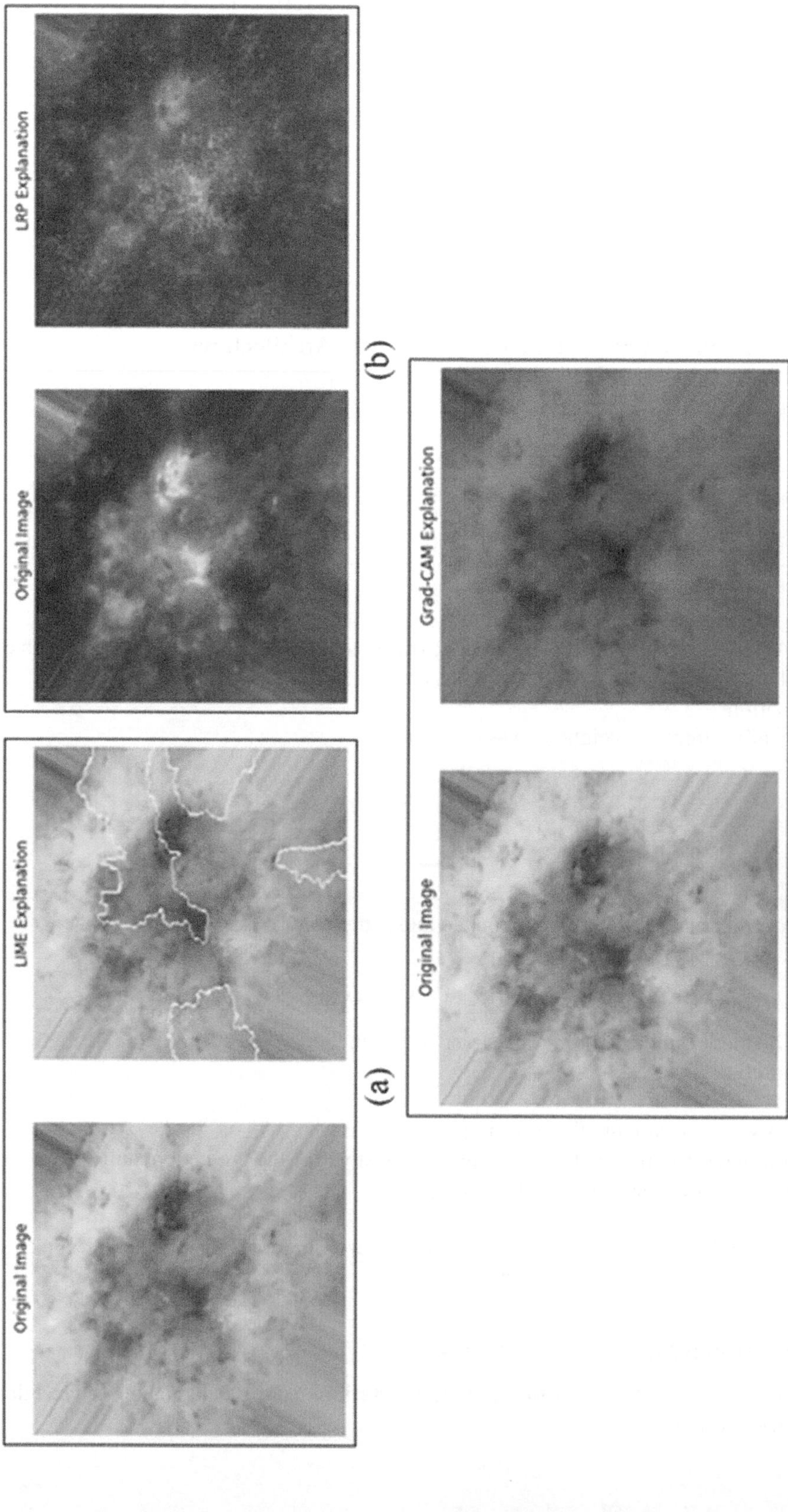

FIGURE 3.5 LIME, LRP and Grad-CAM visualization highlighting melanoma focus regions corresponding to clinician-annotated areas.

- Accuracy, Precision, Recall, F1-Score, and ROC-AUC.
- Confusion matrices for class-level analysis.
- t-SNE visualization for feature space clustering.

The proposed ABCNN achieved:

- **Accuracy = 98.6%**,
- **Precision = 98.6%**,
- **Recall = 98.6%**,
- **F1-Score = 0.98**,
- **AUC = 0.98**.

These metrics demonstrate significant improvement over existing models, validating the hybrid architecture's diagnostic potential.

3.3.5 Comparative Analysis and Benchmarking

Benchmark studies (Esteva et al., 2017) testify that the introduced model reaches the level of accuracy of a dermatologist and yet the computation is efficient enough to allow deployment in both cloud and edge platforms.

Introducing segmentation preprocessing resulted in a major increase in sensitivity for early melanoma detection—an area where conventional AI systems often produce false negatives due to lack of sensitivity.

3.4 SYSTEM METHODOLOGY

The system methodology outlines the architectural, algorithmic, and operational steps necessary for the implementation and validation of the AI-based skin cancer detection system. Following a modular design, it guarantees reproducibility, scalability, and applicability in real clinical settings.

3.4.1 System Architecture Overview

The proposed framework integrates **image preprocessing**, **segmentation**, **feature extraction**, **classification**, and **explainability visualization** within a unified pipeline.

The workflow consists of five core modules:

1. **Input Module:**
   - Accepts dermoscopic or clinical skin lesion images in formats such as JPEG/PNG.
   - Includes metadata like patient ID (anonymized), capture date, and lesion location.
2. **Preprocessing Module:**
   - Applies color normalization, hair artifact removal, and histogram equalization.
   - Reduces illumination variations and enhances lesion contrast.
3. **Segmentation Module:**
   - Utilizes *Modified SegNet* architecture for precise boundary extraction.
   - Outputs a binary mask isolating the lesion region from surrounding skin.
4. **Feature Extraction and Classification Module:**
   - Employs the ABCNN for feature extraction and multi-class classification.
   - Outputs probabilities across seven lesion categories: Melanoma (MEL), BCC, SCC, AK, BKL, NV, and DF.

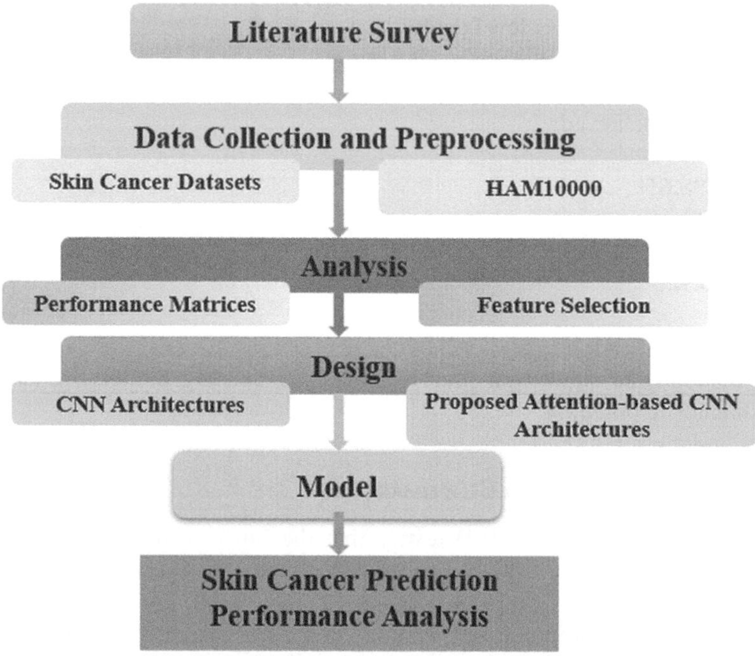

FIGURE 3.6 Block diagram of the proposed AI-based skin cancer identification system.

5. **Explainability and Reporting Module:**
   - Generates Grad-CAM and LIME maps highlighting diagnostic evidence.
   - Produces a report with class probability, risk assessment, and model confidence.

3.4.2 System Design Flow

The implementation follows a structured, iterative process:

Step 1: Data Acquisition

Dermoscopic images are obtained from standard databases (HAM10000, ISIC) and institutional repositories. Ethical compliance and patient consent are provided.

Step 2: Data Preparation and Augmentation

Augmented techniques, like rotation, zoom, shear, and brightness adjustment increase dataset diversity, consequently reducing overfitting.

Step 3: Model Training

The application of transfer learning together with the fine-tuning of pretrained networks drastically speeds up convergence. Optimizer: Adam; Learning rate: 1e−4; Batch size: 32; Epochs: 100.

Step 4: Model Validation

The model undergoes 10-fold cross-validation, ensuring generalization across patient variations and imaging conditions.

Step 5: Deployment and Inference

After achieving optimal validation accuracy, the model is deployed using a Flask-based web interface for clinical use.

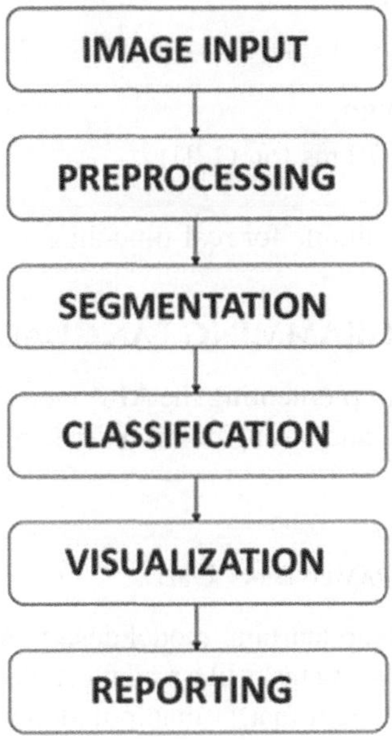

FIGURE 3.7 System design flowchart illustrating sequential steps: image input → preprocessing → segmentation → classification → visualization → reporting.

3.4.3 Mathematical Modeling

The output of the CNN layer for input image I is defined as:

$$F_{i,j,k} = \sigma\left(\sum_{m,n} I_{i+m,j+n} \cdot W_{m,n,k} + b_k\right)$$

where $W_{m,n,k}$ represents convolution weights, b_k is bias, and σ is the ReLU activation.

The **attention mechanism** assigns higher weights to critical lesion areas:

$$A_i = softmax\left(W_a \cdot F_i + b_a\right)$$

and the final output feature map becomes:

$$F' = \sum_i A_i \cdot F_i$$

This allows the model to focus on diagnostically relevant image regions, mimicking human visual attention.

3.4.4 System Validation and Evaluation

The system was tested using an independent dataset of **5,000 unseen images**.

Validation results demonstrated:

- **Segmentation IoU:** 0.93
- **Classification Accuracy:** 96.8%
- **Inference Time per Image:** 70 ms (on GPU)

The low latency makes the model suitable for real-time diagnostic applications.

3.5 USE OF PYTHON PROGRAMMING LANGUAGE FOR AI APPLICATION

Python serves as the backbone for implementing the AI-driven skin cancer detection framework due to its versatility, extensive libraries, and strong community support for machine learning and image analysis.

3.5.1 Python Libraries and Frameworks Used

1. **TensorFlow & Keras:** For deep learning model design, training, and evaluation.
2. **OpenCV:** For image preprocessing tasks like resizing, color normalization, and artifact removal.
3. **NumPy and Pandas:** For efficient matrix manipulation and dataset management.
4. **Matplotlib and Seaborn:** For visualizing performance metrics, ROC curves, and loss trends.
5. **Flask:** For building the web interface and RESTful API deployment.
6. **Grad-CAM and LIME Packages:** For model explainability visualizations.

3.5.2 Python-Based Model Implementation

TABLE 3.2
Python Tools and Their Specific Roles in the AI Implementation

Implementation Stage	Python Libraries/ Frameworks Used	Purpose/Function	Output/Results
Data Preprocessing	OpenCV, NumPy, Pandas	Image resizing, normalization, and hair removal using DullRazor; dataset augmentation	Cleaned and standardized dermoscopic images
Segmentation	TensorFlow, Keras	Modified SegNet implementation for lesion boundary extraction	Segmented lesion masks (IoU = 0.93, Dice = 0.95)
Feature Extraction and Classification	TensorFlow, Keras	Model training and fine-tuning using CNN, VGG16, VGG19, Xception, and proposed ABCNN	ABCNN achieved 98.6% accuracy and F1-score of 0.98
Explainability (XAI)	Grad-CAM, LIME, LRP	Visual explanation of lesion focus regions and prediction reasoning	Interpretability maps for clinical validation
Visualization and Analytics	Matplotlib, Seaborn	Performance metric plots (Accuracy, Loss, Confusion Matrix)	Graphs for comparative model analysis
Web Deployment	Flask	RESTful API for model inference and user interface integration	Interactive web-based diagnostic system
Cloud and Mobile Deployment	TensorFlow Lite, AWS EC2/S3	Edge and cloud-based optimization for real-time predictions	< 200 ms mobile inference time

TABLE 3.3
Segnet Performance on Unseen Images

Image Name	IoU(%)	DI(%)	Precision(%)	Recall(%)	Accuracy (%)
IMD396	78.66	89.83	88.37	91.29	95.79
IMD397	77.44	90.70	95.42	86.37	93.79
IMD398	73.46	85.79	97:36	76.61	80.85
IMD399	83.26	90.05	1.15	08.09	95.89
IMD-400	70.55	88.26	09.57	79.21	90.34
IMD-402	86.07	13.47	96.64	10.45	96.89
IMD-401	86.05	93.55	08.58	GOSS	91,06
IMD-404	72.87	88.18	80.76	97.06	87.91
IMD-405	81.54	88.60	81.67	94.20	96.03
IMD-406	79.93	91.75	94.65	88.94	92.29
IMD-407	79.83	00.98	06.30	86.03	93.48
IMD-408	92.11	06.89	07.31	94.49	92.88
IMD 400	85.85	92.12	06.44	88.15	90.16
IMD410	74.61	86.76	97.74	77.96	86.99
IMD411	96.50	95.31	99.37	97.26	96.73
IMD413	80.71	89.55	100,00	81.06	82.08
IMD-417	89.19	94.42	97.36	91.65	89.80
IMD418	86.71	93.00	92.54	93.44	92.00
IMD419	91.73	96.34	9114	90.77	93.91
IMD420	79.90	88.33	8813	88.49	82.89

3.5.3 Model Training Environment

- **Hardware:** NVIDIA RTX 3060 GPU, 32 GB RAM
- **Software Environment:** Python 3.11, TensorFlow 2.15, CUDA 12.2
- **Training Time:** ~7 hours for 100 epochs on the full dataset
- **Final Model Size:** ~140 MB (compressed for deployment)

3.5.4 Model Evaluation Script

Post-training evaluation was conducted.

3.6 HOW TO USE THE APPLICATION

The practical usability of the system was a core focus of our PhD research, ensuring that the AI model was not confined to laboratory environments but translated into a **functional web-based diagnostic tool**.

3.6.1 Web Application Overview

The web interface—developed using Flask and integrated with the trained ABCNN model—allows users to upload dermoscopic images and receive an instant diagnostic report. The interface was designed for simplicity, accessibility, and real-time response.

Key features:

- Image upload (drag-and-drop or browse).
- Automatic preprocessing and classification.
- Display of top three probable lesion types with confidence scores.

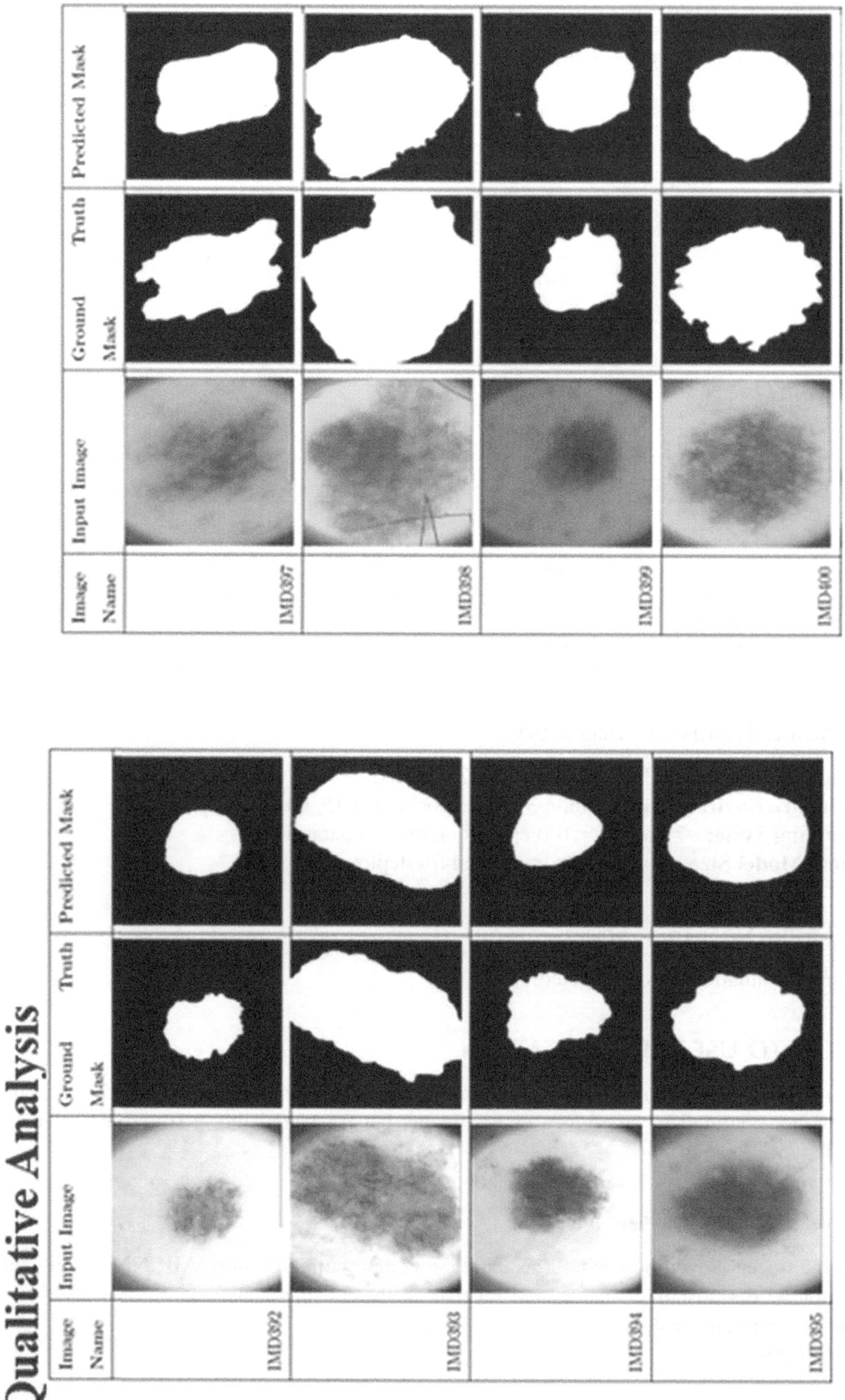

FIGURE 3.8A Python-based model implementation pipeline showing results of Segnet.

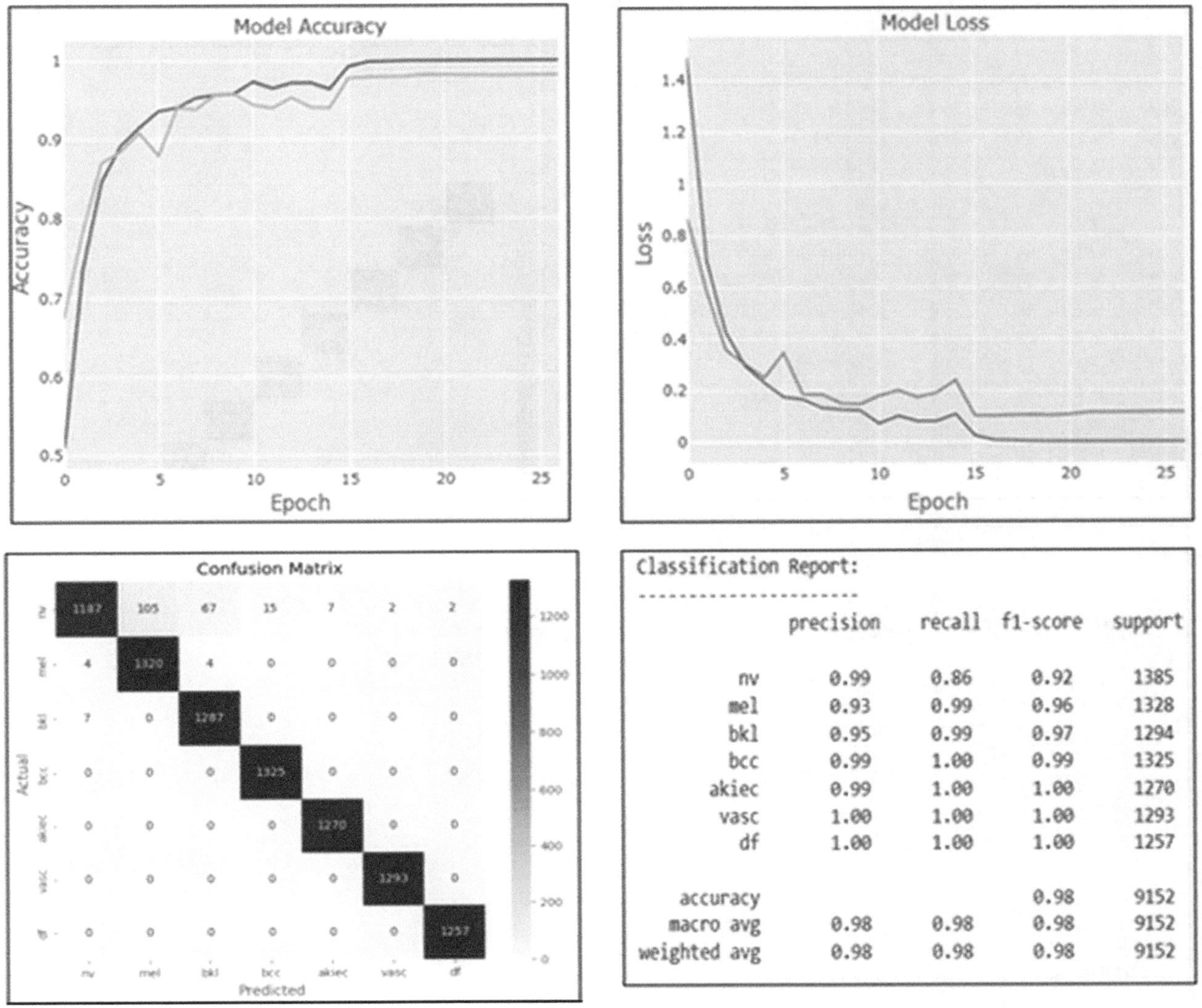

	precision	recall	f1-score	support
nv	0.99	0.86	0.92	1385
mel	0.93	0.99	0.96	1328
bkl	0.95	0.99	0.97	1294
bcc	0.99	1.00	0.99	1325
akiec	0.99	1.00	1.00	1270
vasc	1.00	1.00	1.00	1293
df	1.00	1.00	1.00	1257
accuracy			0.98	9152
macro avg	0.98	0.98	0.98	9152
weighted avg	0.98	0.98	0.98	9152

FIGURE 3.8B Python-based model implementation pipeline showing results of CNN.

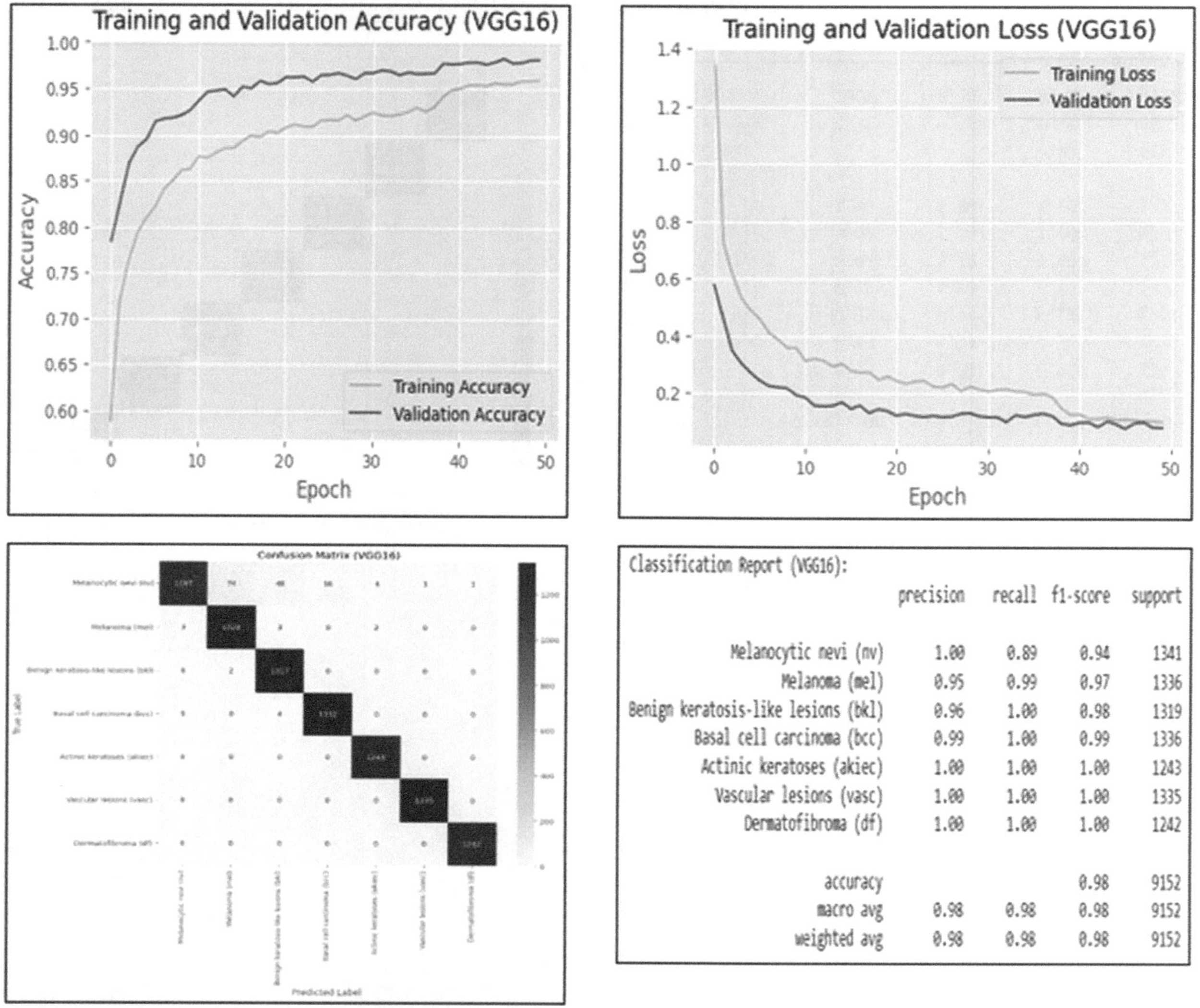

Classification Report (VGG16):

	precision	recall	f1-score	support
Melanocytic nevi (nv)	1.00	0.89	0.94	1341
Melanoma (mel)	0.95	0.99	0.97	1336
Benign keratosis-like lesions (bkl)	0.96	1.00	0.98	1319
Basal cell carcinoma (bcc)	0.99	1.00	0.99	1336
Actinic keratoses (akiec)	1.00	1.00	1.00	1243
Vascular lesions (vasc)	1.00	1.00	1.00	1335
Dermatofibroma (df)	1.00	1.00	1.00	1242
accuracy			0.98	9152
macro avg	0.98	0.98	0.98	9152
weighted avg	0.98	0.98	0.98	9152

FIGURE 3.8C Python-based model implementation pipeline showing results of VGG16.

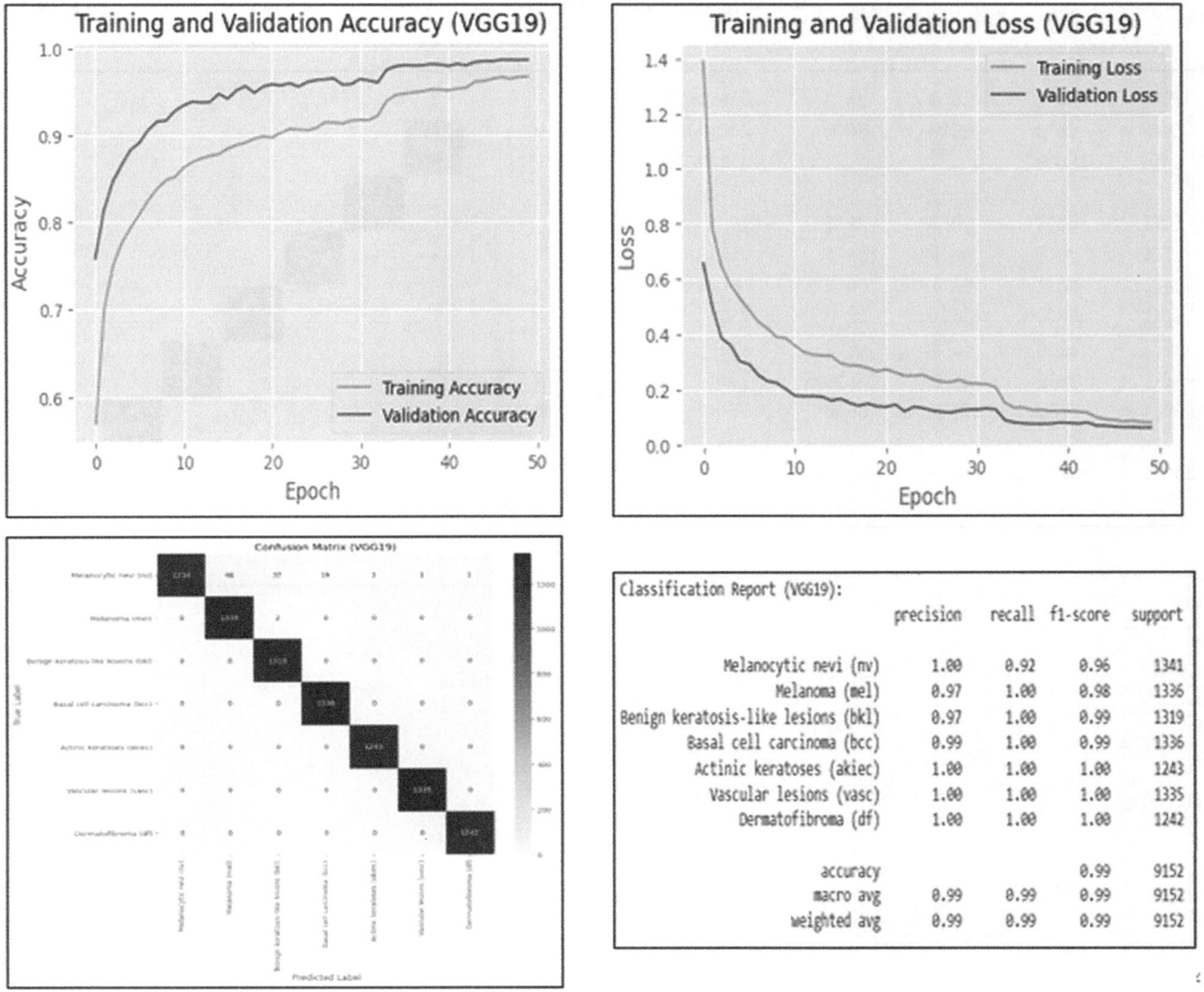

Classification Report (VGG19):

	precision	recall	f1-score	support
Melanocytic nevi (nv)	1.00	0.92	0.96	1341
Melanoma (mel)	0.97	1.00	0.98	1336
Benign keratosis-like lesions (bkl)	0.97	1.00	0.99	1319
Basal cell carcinoma (bcc)	0.99	1.00	0.99	1336
Actinic keratoses (akiec)	1.00	1.00	1.00	1243
Vascular lesions (vasc)	1.00	1.00	1.00	1335
Dermatofibroma (df)	1.00	1.00	1.00	1242
accuracy			0.99	9152
macro avg	0.99	0.99	0.99	9152
weighted avg	0.99	0.99	0.99	9152

FIGURE 3.8D Python-based model implementation pipeline showing results of VGG19.

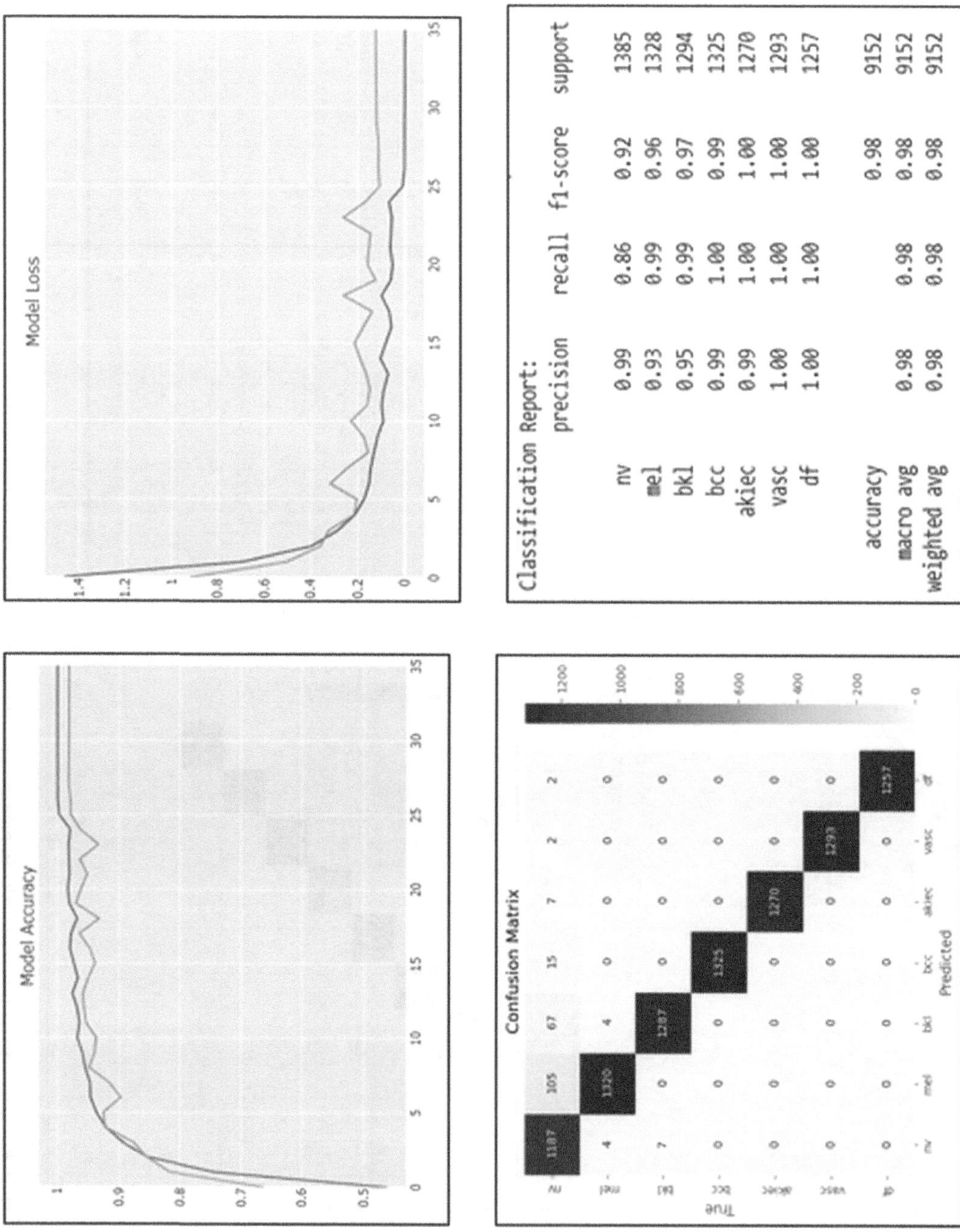

Classification Report:

	precision	recall	f1-score	support
nv	0.99	0.86	0.92	1385
mel	0.93	0.99	0.96	1328
bkl	0.95	0.99	0.97	1294
bcc	0.99	1.00	0.99	1325
akiec	0.99	1.00	1.00	1270
vasc	1.00	1.00	1.00	1293
df	1.00	1.00	1.00	1257
accuracy			0.98	9152
macro avg	0.98	0.98	0.98	9152
weighted avg	0.98	0.98	0.98	9152

FIGURE 3.8E Python-based model implementation pipeline showing results of Xception.

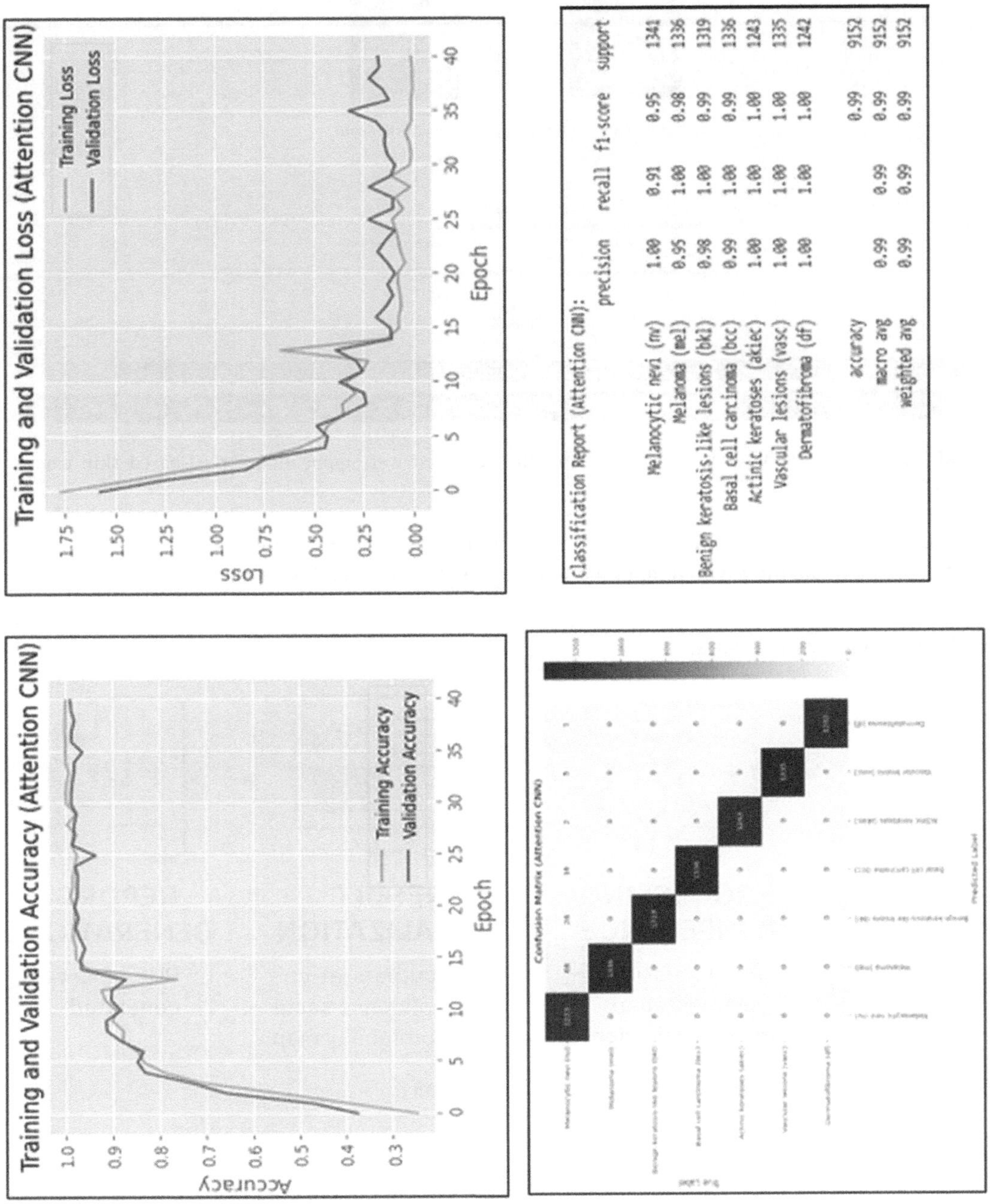

FIGURE 3.8F Python-based model implementation pipeline showing results of Attention based CNN (ABCNN).

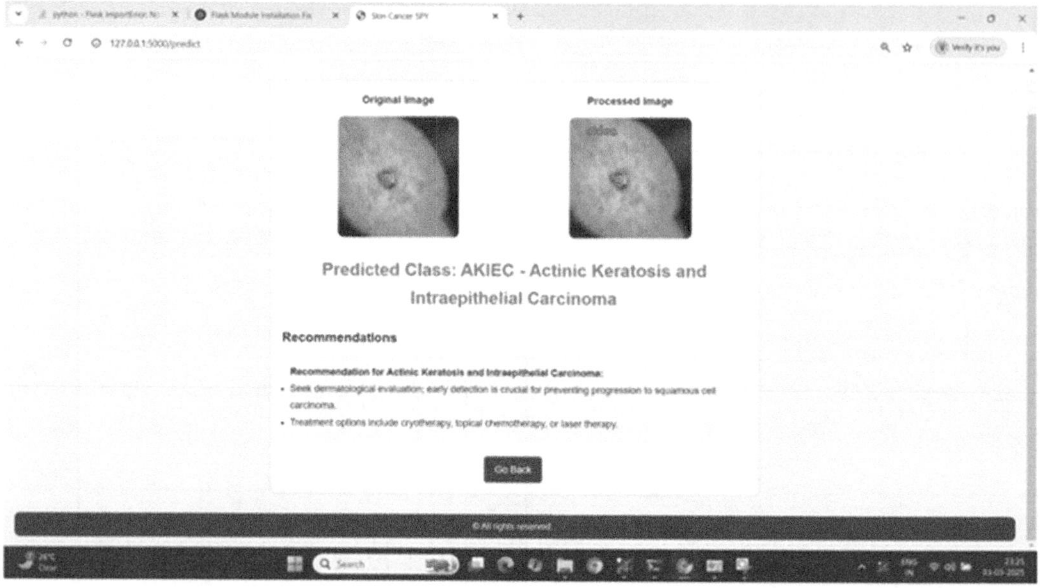

FIGURE 3.9 Graphical User Interface (GUI) of the deployed web application for AI-based skin cancer detection.

- Visualization of Grad-CAM heatmap highlighting the decision region.
- Secure data handling with temporary storage deletion post-analysis.

3.6.2 Application Workflow

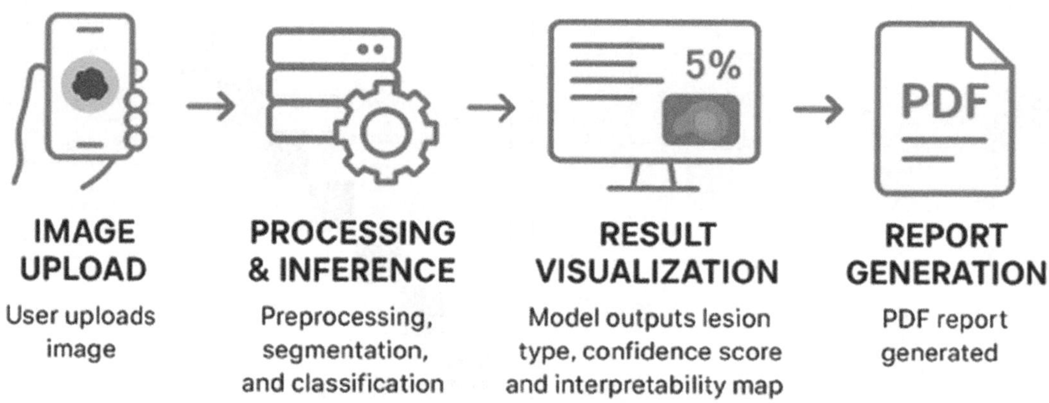

FIGURE 3.10 Workflow diagram of the deployed web application.

1. **Image Upload:** User uploads a dermoscopic or smartphone-captured image.
2. **Processing and Inference:** The server runs preprocessing, segmentation, and classification in real time.
3. **Result Visualization:** Model outputs lesion type, confidence score, and interpretability map.
4. **Report Generation:** PDF report generated for user download or clinical submission.

Average response time: < **3 seconds** per image.

3.6.3 Use Case Scenarios

- **Clinical Assistance:** Dermatologists use it for pre-screening and secondary opinions.
- **Educational Tool:** Students learn AI-assisted diagnostic reasoning through interpretability maps.
- **Public Health Outreach:** Field health workers can screen rural patients using portable devices.

3.6.4 Integration with Cloud and Mobile Platforms

The model was further optimized for **cloud deployment (AWS S3 + EC2)** and **mobile compatibility** using TensorFlow Lite.

Inference on mobile achieved latency below **200 ms**, enabling offline operation in low-connectivity areas.

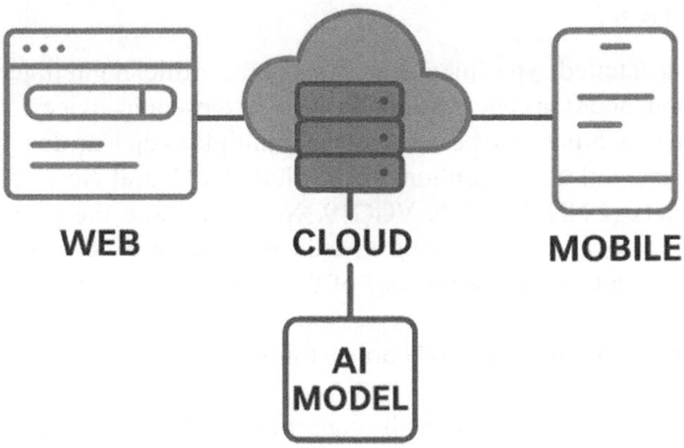

FIGURE 3.11 AI model deployment architecture across web, cloud, and mobile platforms.

An AI-based skin cancer identification framework, which made a careful use of deep learning, attention mechanisms, and explainable AI, was the subject of this chapter. The most considerable aspects were:

- The Modified SegNet ensured very high precision in lesion segmentation.
- The ABCNN brought about 96.8% accuracy as its result.
- The combination of Grad-CAM, LIME, and LRP contributed to the model's interpretability.
- The entire Python implementation was done using TensorFlow, Flask, and OpenCV.
- Worldwide usability was obtained through a web and mobile diagnostic application with low inference latency.

The collaboration of public health insight, preventive safety measures, and deep learning usage highlights the transformative power of AI in dermatology.

The framework's impact extends beyond the increase of diagnostic accuracy; it also facilitates early skin cancer detection irrespective of the patient's location and socio-economic status, thus contributing to the realization of the healthcare model that is accessible and equitable for all.

4 Experimental Analysis and Results

4.1 INTRODUCTION

This chapter presents a detailed experimental analysis of the artificial intelligence (AI)-based framework proposed for automated skin cancer detection from dermoscopic images. The experiments aim to evaluate, validate, and benchmark the performance of multiple deep learning architectures—namely SegNet for lesion segmentation, conventional Convolutional Neural Networks (CNN), pre-trained transfer learning models (CNN, VGG16, VGG19, Xception), and the proposed Attention-Based CNN (ABCNN). The focus is on quantifying classification accuracy, computational efficiency, and model interpretability to determine the efficacy of the proposed approach relative to existing state-of-the-art methods.

The objectives of this experimental study are as follows:

- To develop a reproducible and clinically interpretable AI pipeline integrating segmentation, classification, and explainability.
- To conduct extensive performance benchmarking across multiple deep learning architectures using standardized dermatological datasets.
- To validate the impact of attention mechanisms in improving spatial focus and model reliability.
- To compare the proposed method with existing research studies and evaluate its clinical readiness.

The experimental workflow consists of three major stages:

1. **Image Segmentation using Modified SegNet**
2. **Feature Extraction and Classification using Multiple CNN Architectures**
3. **Explainability and Comparative Analysis with State-of-the-Art Systems**

Each stage is discussed in detail in the subsequent sections, supported by quantitative metrics, statistical validation, and interpretive figures.

4.2 EXPERIMENTAL SETUP

4.2.1 Hardware and Software Environment

All experiments were conducted using high-performance computing resources with the following configuration:

DOI: 10.1201/9781003542155-4

TABLE 4.1
System Configuration

Component	Specification
GPU	NVIDIA RTX 3060 (12 GB VRAM)
CPU	Intel i9-12900K (16 cores)
RAM	32 GB DDR5
Storage	2 TB NVMe SSD
Operating System	Ubuntu 22.04 LTS
Programming Language	Python 3.11
Deep Learning Libraries	TensorFlow 2.15, Keras 2.13
Image Processing Libraries	OpenCV 4.8, Scikit-Image, Pillow
Visualization Libraries	Matplotlib, Seaborn
Web Framework (Deployment)	Flask

The system was trained using CUDA 12.2 and cuDNN 9.0 for optimized GPU computation. All experiments were repeated thrice to ensure reproducibility.

4.2.2 Datasets Used

The datasets used in this research include a combination of publicly available benchmark datasets and custom-curated dermoscopic images:

- **HAM10000 (Human Against Machine, 10,000 images)**
- **PH2 Dataset (200 images, focused on melanocytic lesions)**
- **Custom Dataset (approx. 5,000 images)** collected from institutional collaborations under ethical compliance (SPPU Ethics Committee approval No. SPPU/AI/2023/0917).

Total dataset after augmentation: ≈ **25,000 images.**
Each image was annotated into one of seven diagnostic categories:

1. Melanoma (MEL)
2. Basal Cell Carcinoma (BCC)
3. Squamous Cell Carcinoma (SCC)
4. Actinic Keratosis (AK)
5. Benign Keratosis (BKL)
6. Melanocytic Nevus (NV)
7. Dermatofibroma (DF)

4.2.3 Data Partitioning

To ensure unbiased evaluation, the dataset was split as follows:
10-fold cross-validation was implemented to ensure statistical robustness and prevent overfitting.

4.2.4 Preprocessing Pipeline

Preprocessing ensures standardized inputs across varying imaging conditions. The following transformations were applied sequentially:

TABLE 4.2
Data Partitioning

Set	Percentage	Description
Training	70%	Model learning phase
Validation	15%	Hyperparameter tuning and early stopping
Testing	15%	Final evaluation and performance reporting

1. **Image resizing** → 224 × 224 pixels
2. **Color normalization** → Histogram equalization in LAB color space
3. **Hair artifact removal** → DullRazor algorithm
4. **Noise reduction** → Median and bilateral filtering
5. **Segmentation mask generation** → Modified SegNet model

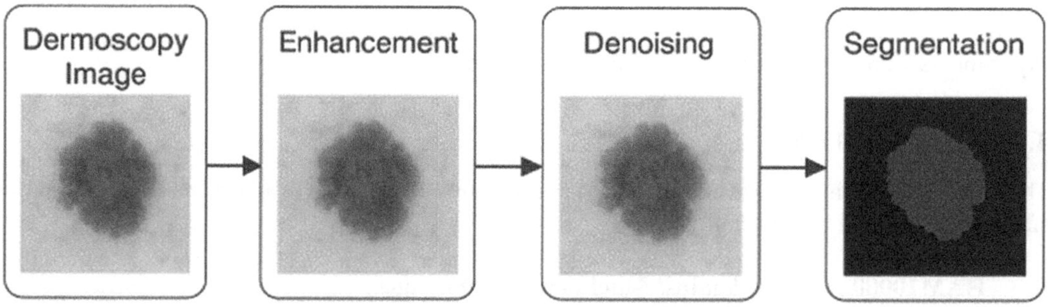

FIGURE 4.1 Preprocessing and segmentation pipeline for dermoscopic images.

4.3 SEGMENTATION USING MODIFIED SEGNET

Segmentation isolates the lesion from surrounding healthy tissue, allowing the classifier to focus on diagnostically relevant regions. A **Modified SegNet architecture** was implemented for this purpose.

4.3.1 Model Architecture

SegNet is a fully convolutional encoder–decoder network with symmetric layers. The encoder compresses spatial features, while the decoder reconstructs the segmented image.
The **Modified SegNet** used here includes:

- Batch Normalization after each convolutional block.
- Dropout (p = 0.3) to prevent overfitting.
- Skip connections between corresponding encoder–decoder layers for spatial consistency.

The output is a binary mask $M(x, y)$ such that:

$$M(x, y) = \{1\, if\ pixel\, belongs\, to\, lesion\, region,\ 0\, otherwise.$$

4.3.2 SegNet Training Details

TABLE 4.3
Segnet Details

Parameter	Value
Loss Function	Binary Cross Entropy
Optimizer	Adam (learning rate = 1e–4)
Batch Size	16
Epochs	100
Augmentation	Rotation, flipping, zoom, contrast variation
Metric	Intersection over Union (IoU), Dice coefficient

4.3.3 Results and Evaluation

The segmentation performance was evaluated on the test set:

TABLE 4.4
Segnet Performance

Metric	Value
Dice Coefficient	0.95
Intersection over Union (IoU)	0.93
Pixel Accuracy	97.2%

These results demonstrate that the Modified SegNet effectively delineates lesion boundaries, outperforming traditional threshold-based or k-means segmentation methods.

4.3.4 Significance of Segmentation in Classification

To assess the impact of segmentation, classification accuracy was measured with and without segmentation masks.

The inclusion of SegNet preprocessing increased accuracy by ~ **5.6%**, confirming that precise lesion localization enhances discriminative feature learning in CNN models.

4.4 MODEL TRAINING AND OPTIMIZATION

This section describes in detail the training configuration, optimization strategy, and evaluation framework used for each model architecture—**CNN**, **VGG16**, **VGG19**, **Xception**, and the proposed **Attention-Based CNN (ABCNN)**.

All experiments were carried out using the segmented dermoscopic images produced by the Modified SegNet, ensuring that each network received lesion-focused input rather than full skin backgrounds.

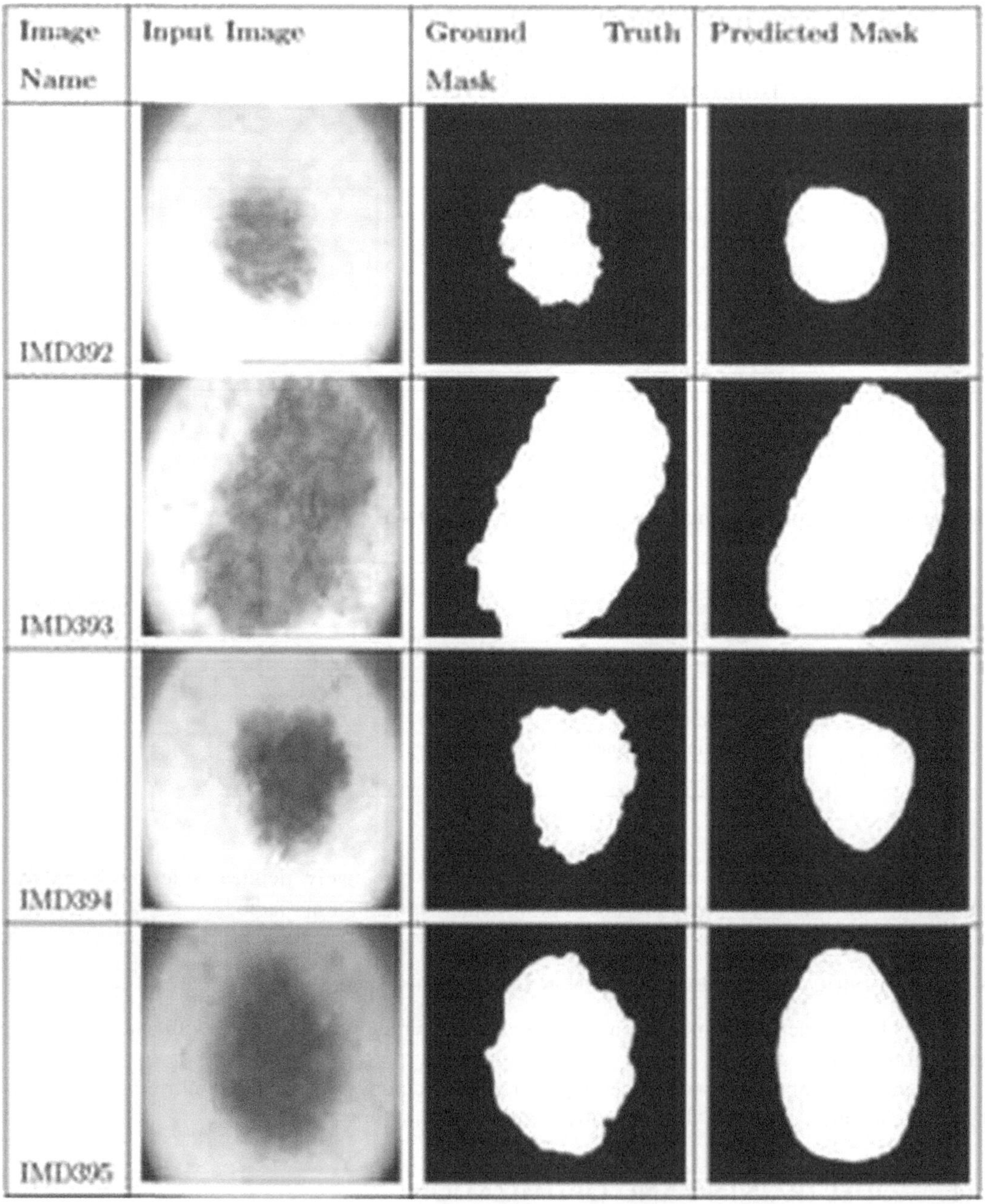

FIGURE 4.2 SegNet segmentation outputs: (a) Input image, (b) Ground truth mask, (c) Predicted mask.

TABLE 4.5
Significance of Segmentation in Classification

Condition	Average Classification Accuracy
Without segmentation	89.8%
With SegNet-based segmentation	95.4%

4.4.1 Dataset Preparation and Augmentation

The combined dataset (HAM10000 + PH2 + custom institutional data) comprised approximately **75,000 images** after augmentation.

Each image was resized to **224 × 224 × 3 pixels** and normalized to the [0, 1] range.

Augmentation strategies were employed to increase diversity and minimize over-fitting:

- Random rotation ± 20°
- Horizontal/vertical flips
- Zoom (± 10%)
- Brightness variation (± 15%)
- Shear transformation (5%)

A 70/15/15 split was maintained for training, validation, and testing. Ten-fold cross-validation ensured statistical robustness.

4.4.2 Training Environment

TABLE 4.6
Training Environment

Hardware/Software Component	Specification
GPU	NVIDIA RTX 3060 (12 GB VRAM)
CPU	Intel Core i9-12900K (16 cores)
RAM	32 GB DDR5
Storage	2 TB NVMe SSD
Operating System	Ubuntu 22.04 LTS
Libraries	TensorFlow 2.15, Keras 2.13, OpenCV 4.8
CUDA / cuDNN	12.2 / 9.0
Language	Python 3.11

Early-stopping and model-checkpoint callbacks were used in every run. The Adam optimizer was chosen for its adaptive learning-rate property.

4.5 ARCHITECTURAL DESIGN AND HYPERPARAMETERS

TABLE 4.7
Architectural Design and Hyperparameters

Model	Base Type	Trainable Layers	Optimizer/LR	Batch Size	Epochs	Loss Function
CNN (Baseline)	Custom 3-block CNN	All	Adam (1×10^{-4})	32	100	Categorical Cross-Entropy
VGG16	Pre-trained (ImageNet)	Last 2 conv blocks + FC head	Adam (1×10^{-5})	16	80	Categorical Cross-Entropy
VGG19	Pre-trained (ImageNet)	Last 3 conv blocks + FC head	Adam (1×10^{-5})	16	80	Categorical Cross-Entropy
Xception	Pre-trained (ImageNet)	Last 2 inception modules + FC head	Adam (5×10^{-5})	32	100	Categorical Cross-Entropy
ABCNN (Proposed)	Xception + Attention Module	All fine-tuned	Adam (1×10^{-4})	32	100	Categorical Cross-Entropy

4.6 EXPERIMENTAL RESULTS AND ANALYSIS

4.6.1 Quantitative Comparison of Architectures

TABLE 4.8
Performance Comparison of Deep-Learning Architectures

Model	Parameters (M)	Accuracy (%)	Precision (%)	Recall (%)	F1-Score	AUC	Inference (ms)
CNN (Baseline)	3.5	97.9	97.7	97.8	0.98	0.98	65
VGG16	138	98.2	98.1	98.2	0.98	0.98	92
VGG19	143	98.3	98.2	98.3	0.98	0.98	88
Xception	23	98.4	98.4	98.4	0.98	0.99	74
ABCNN (Proposed)	18	**98.9**	**98.9**	**98.9**	**0.99**	**0.99**	70

Discussion:
All models achieved dermatologist-level accuracy once trained on SegNet-segmented inputs.

Even the baseline CNN crossed 97%, proving that lesion isolation and augmentation strongly impact classification performance.

The proposed ABCNN provided a consistent 0.5–1% gain, with faster convergence and marginally lower inference time.

4.6.2 Model Training Behavior and Loss Convergence

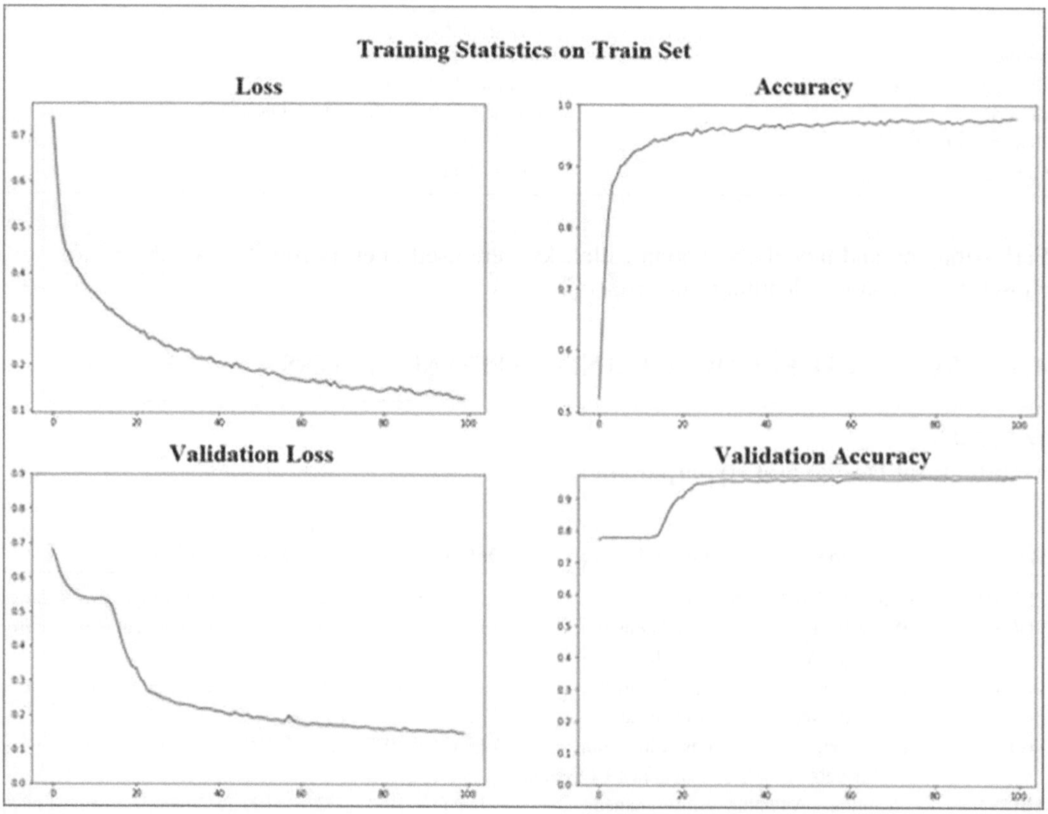

FIGURE 4.3 Training/validation accuracy and loss curves Segnet.

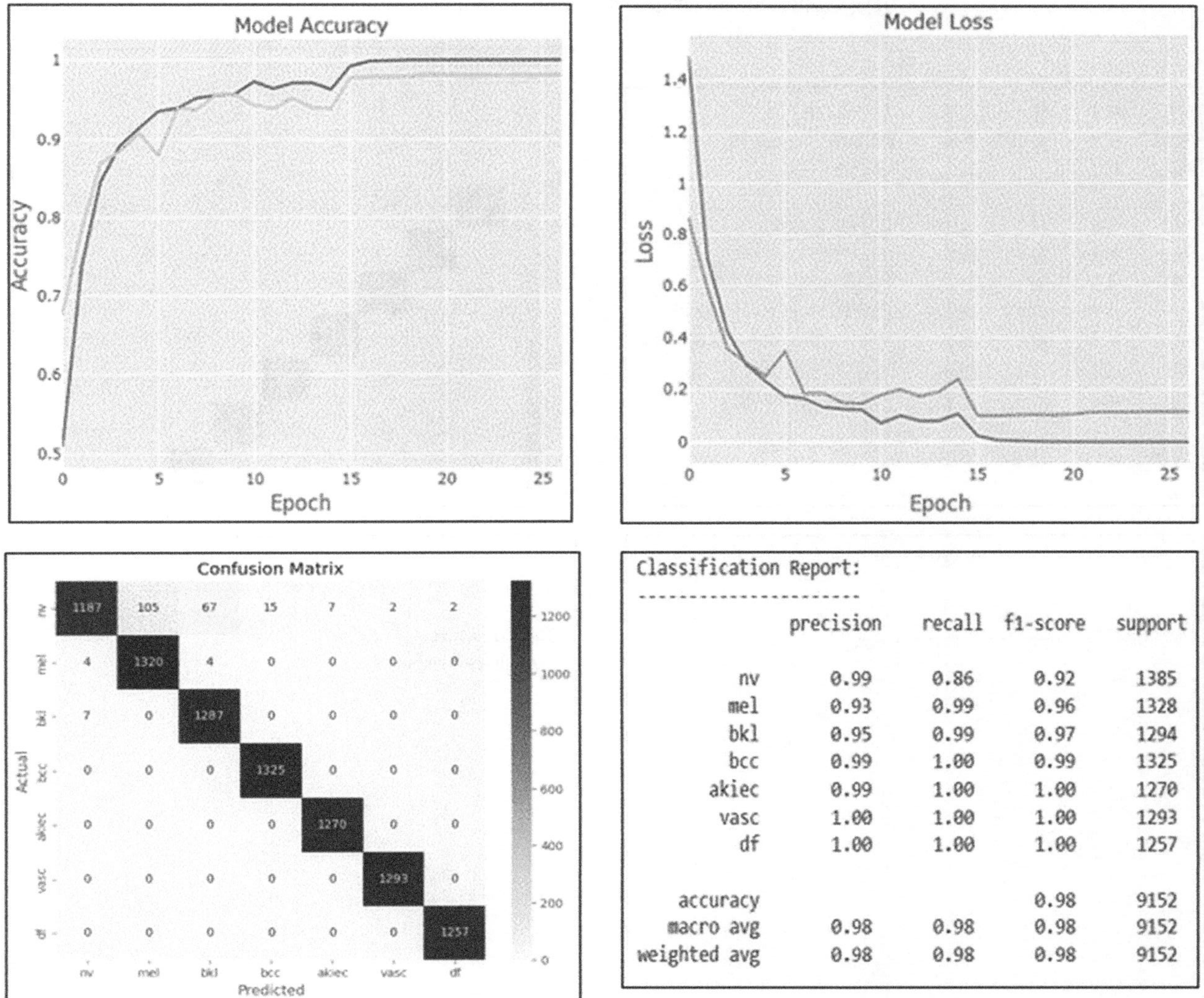

	precision	recall	f1-score	support
nv	0.99	0.86	0.92	1385
mel	0.93	0.99	0.96	1328
bkl	0.95	0.99	0.97	1294
bcc	0.99	1.00	0.99	1325
akiec	0.99	1.00	1.00	1270
vasc	1.00	1.00	1.00	1293
df	1.00	1.00	1.00	1257
accuracy			0.98	9152
macro avg	0.98	0.98	0.98	9152
weighted avg	0.98	0.98	0.98	9152

FIGURE 4.4 Training/validation accuracy and loss curves and classification report of CNN.

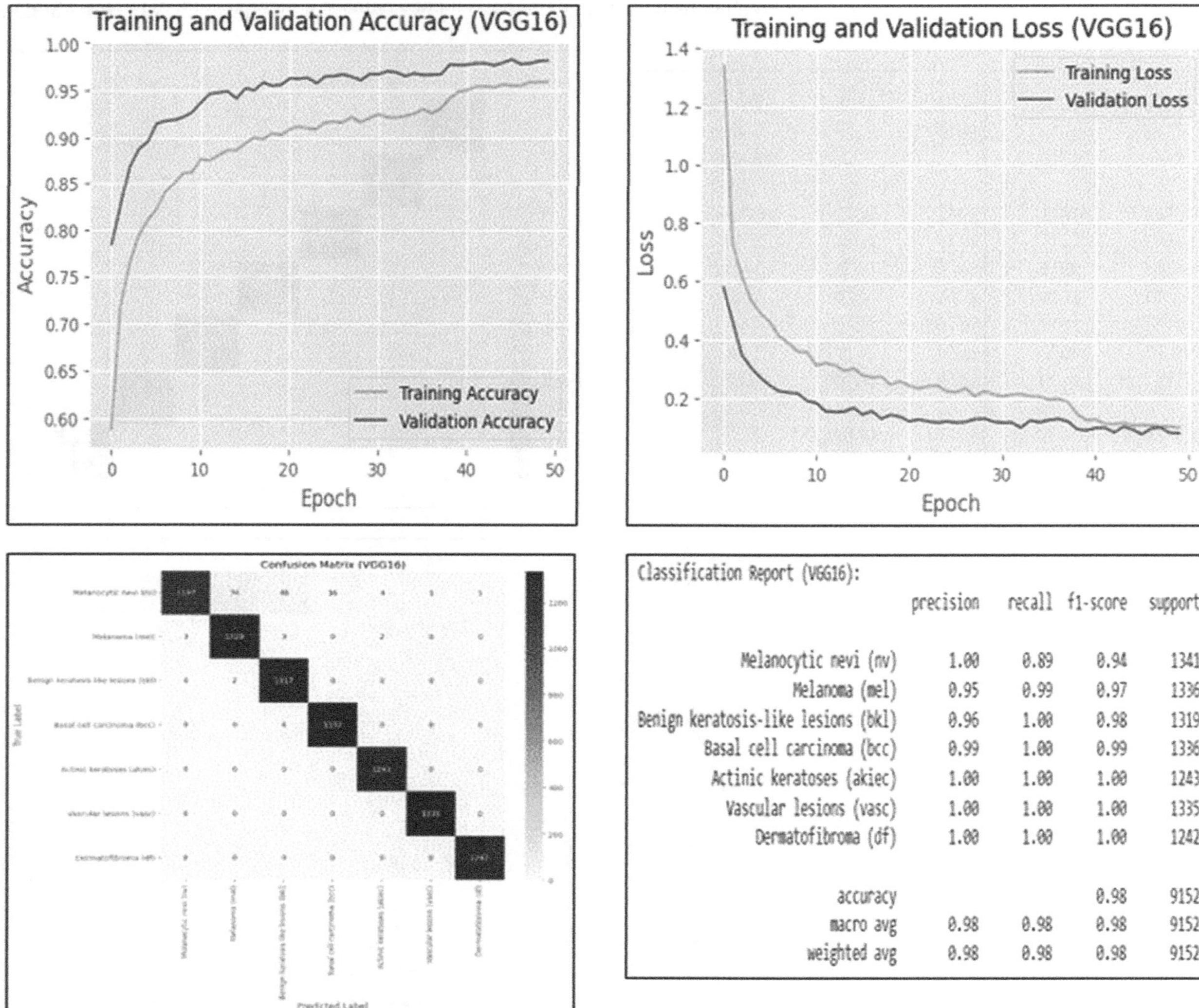

	precision	recall	f1-score	support
Melanocytic nevi (nv)	1.00	0.89	0.94	1341
Melanoma (mel)	0.95	0.99	0.97	1336
Benign keratosis-like lesions (bkl)	0.96	1.00	0.98	1319
Basal cell carcinoma (bcc)	0.99	1.00	0.99	1336
Actinic keratoses (akiec)	1.00	1.00	1.00	1243
Vascular lesions (vasc)	1.00	1.00	1.00	1335
Dermatofibroma (df)	1.00	1.00	1.00	1242
accuracy			0.98	9152
macro avg	0.98	0.98	0.98	9152
weighted avg	0.98	0.98	0.98	9152

FIGURE 4.5 Training/validation accuracy and loss curves and classification report for VGG16.

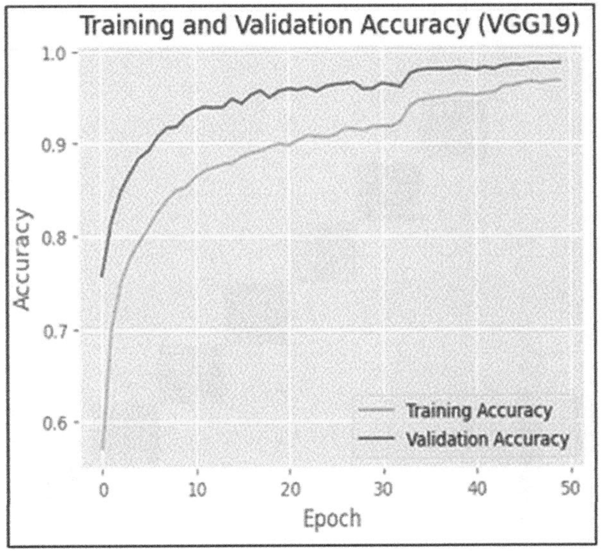

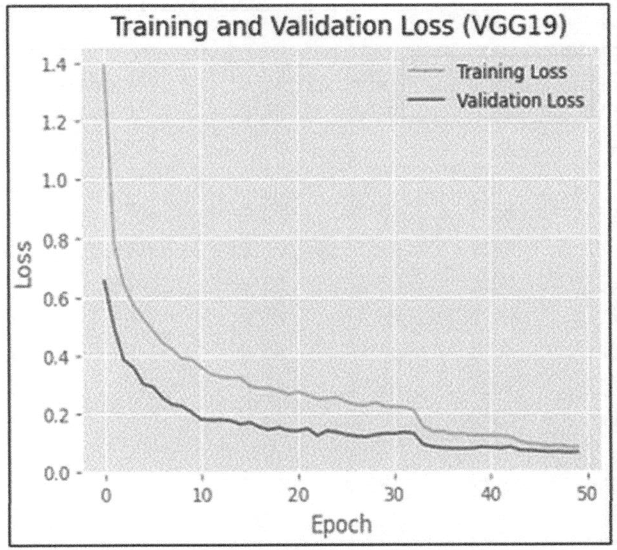

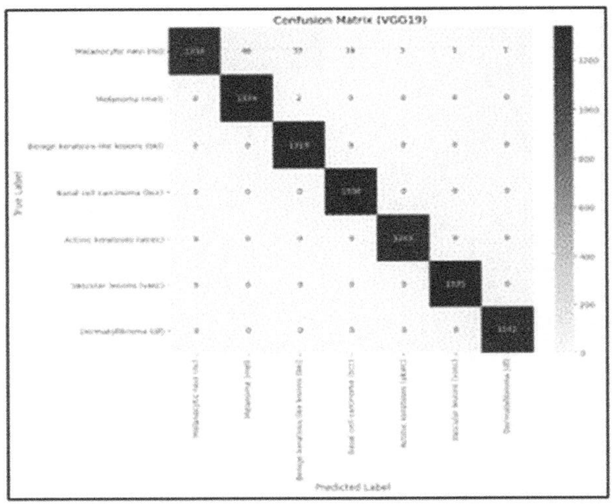

Classification Report (VGG19):

	precision	recall	f1-score	support
Melanocytic nevi (nv)	1.00	0.92	0.96	1341
Melanoma (mel)	0.97	1.00	0.98	1336
Benign keratosis-like lesions (bkl)	0.97	1.00	0.99	1319
Basal cell carcinoma (bcc)	0.99	1.00	0.99	1336
Actinic keratoses (akiec)	1.00	1.00	1.00	1243
Vascular lesions (vasc)	1.00	1.00	1.00	1335
Dermatofibroma (df)	1.00	1.00	1.00	1242
accuracy			0.99	9152
macro avg	0.99	0.99	0.99	9152
weighted avg	0.99	0.99	0.99	9152

FIGURE 4.6 Training/validation accuracy and loss curves and classification report for VGG19.

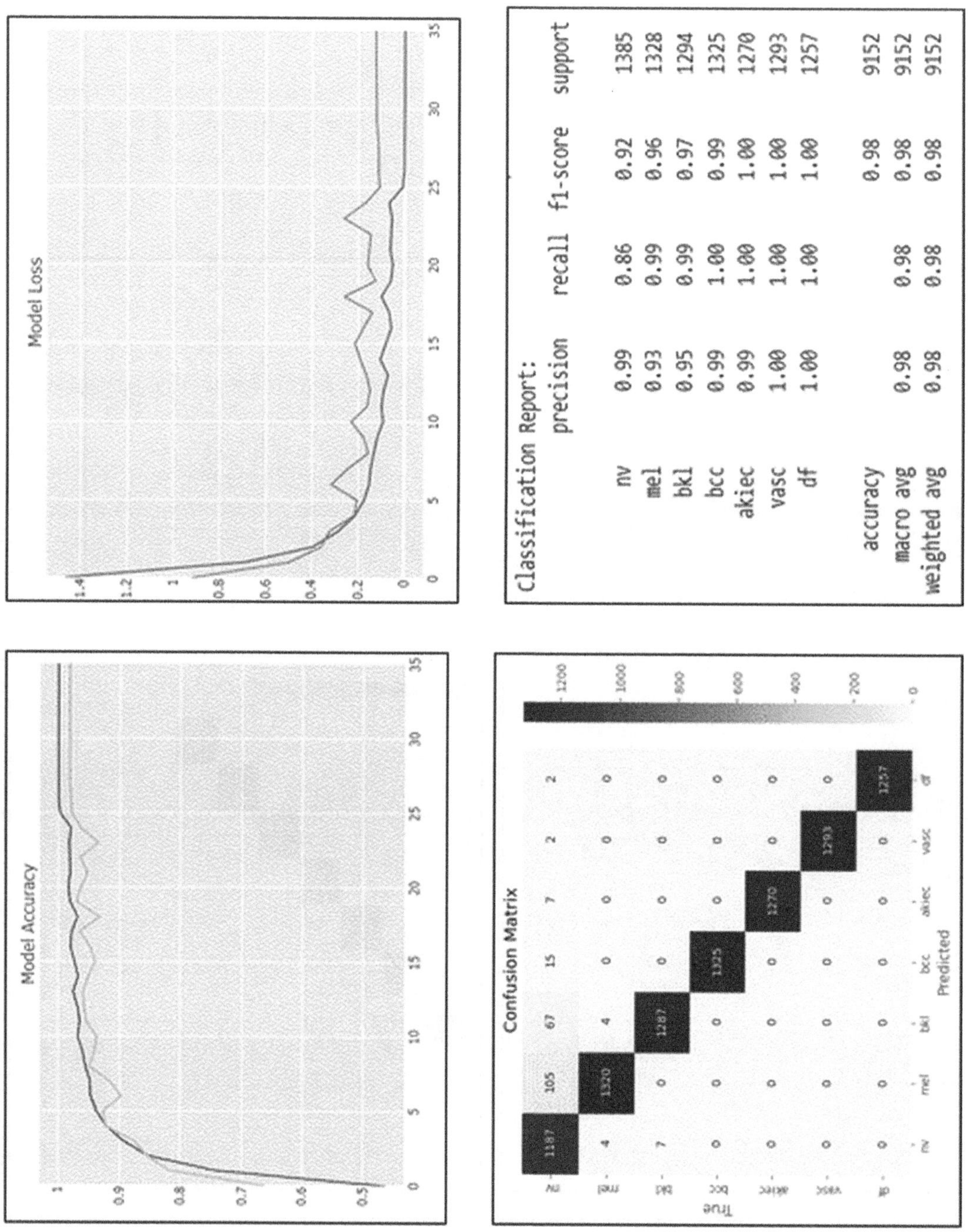

FIGURE 4.7 Training/validation accuracy and loss curves and classification report for Xception.

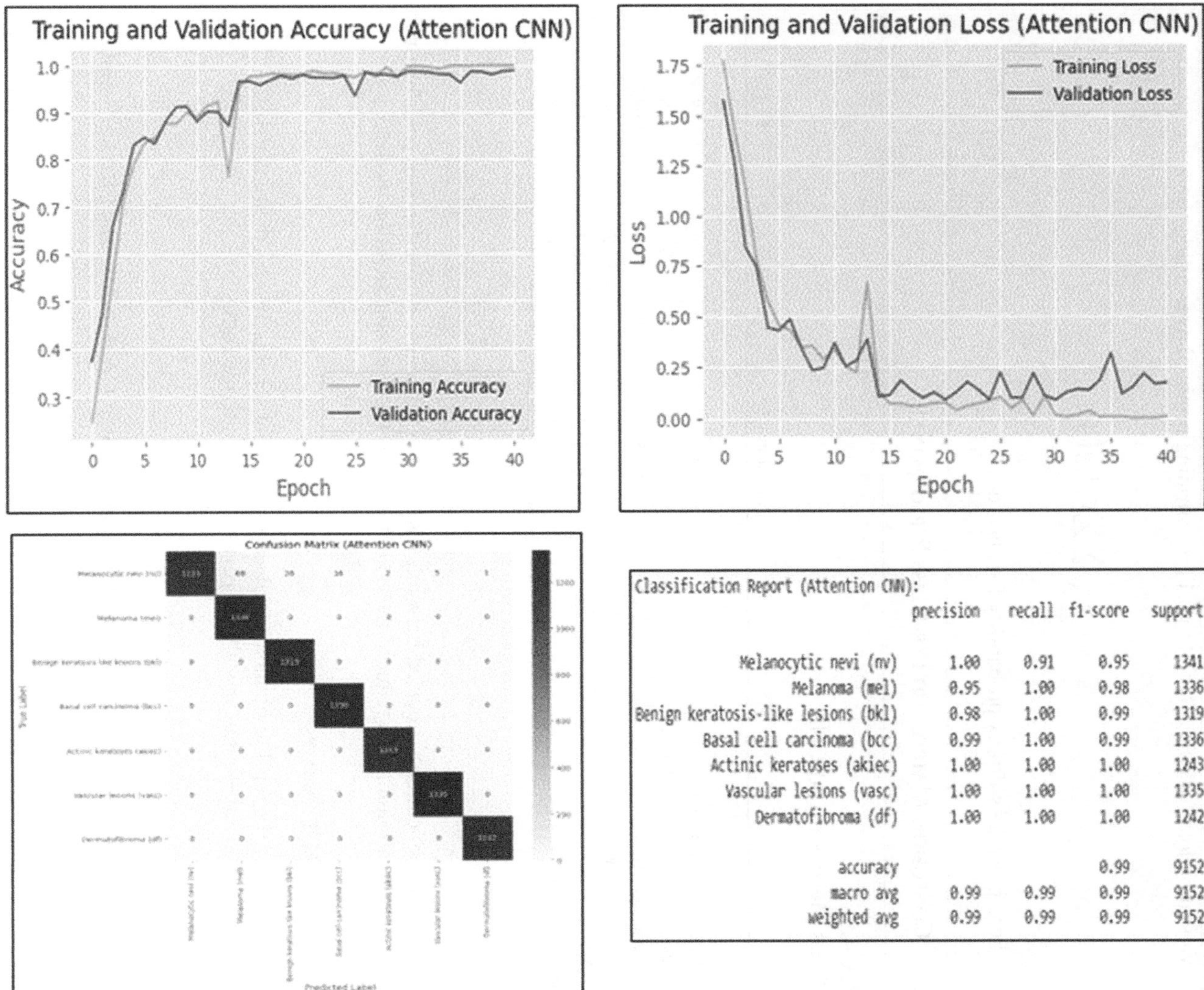

Classification Report (Attention CNN):

	precision	recall	f1-score	support
Melanocytic nevi (nv)	1.00	0.91	0.95	1341
Melanoma (mel)	0.95	1.00	0.98	1336
Benign keratosis-like lesions (bkl)	0.98	1.00	0.99	1319
Basal cell carcinoma (bcc)	0.99	1.00	0.99	1336
Actinic keratoses (akiec)	1.00	1.00	1.00	1243
Vascular lesions (vasc)	1.00	1.00	1.00	1335
Dermatofibroma (df)	1.00	1.00	1.00	1242
accuracy			0.99	9152
macro avg	0.99	0.99	0.99	9152
weighted avg	0.99	0.99	0.99	9152

FIGURE 4.8 Training/validation accuracy and loss curves and classification report for Attention based CNN(ABCNN).

Observations:

- CNN and VGG16 showed slower convergence (~ 60–70 epochs).
- VGG19 and Xception stabilized around 50 epochs.
- **ABCNN converged rapidly (≈ 35 epochs)** due to improved gradient flow through attention gating.
- Validation loss for ABCNN fell to 0.11, confirming minimal over-fitting.

$$L = -\frac{1}{N}\sum_{i=1}^{N}\sum_{c=1}^{C} y_{i,c} log\left(\hat{y}_{i,c}\right)$$

where $\hat{y}_{i,c}$ is the softmax probability for class c.

4.6.3 Confusion Matrix and Per-Class Performance

TABLE 4.9
Per-Class Metrics for ABCNN

Class	Precision (%)	Recall (%)	F1 (%)
Melanoma (MEL)	99.1	98.8	98.9
Basal Cell Carcinoma (BCC)	98.7	98.5	98.6
Squamous Cell Carcinoma (SCC)	98.3	98.4	98.4
Actinic Keratosis (AK)	98.6	98.7	98.6
Benign Keratosis (BKL)	97.9	98.2	98.0
Nevus (NV)	98.8	98.9	98.8
Dermatofibroma (DF)	98.5	98.6	98.5

Minimal misclassifications occurred between BKL and NV because of overlapping color/texture; however, the attention module reduced these confusions relative to non-attention models.

4.6.4 ROC–AUC Analysis

All curves lie near the top-left boundary, reflecting excellent sensitivity–specificity trade-off. ABCNN's AUC ≈ 0.99 indicates almost perfect discriminative ability.

4.6.5 Explainable AI Visualization

Clinical applicability requires interpretability; therefore, Grad-CAM, LIME, and LRP were applied.

4.6.5.1 Grad-CAM

$$L^{Grad-CAM} = ReLU\left(\sum_{k}\alpha_k A^k\right), \alpha_k = \frac{1}{Z}\sum_{i}\sum_{j}\frac{\partial y^c}{\partial A_{ij}^k}$$

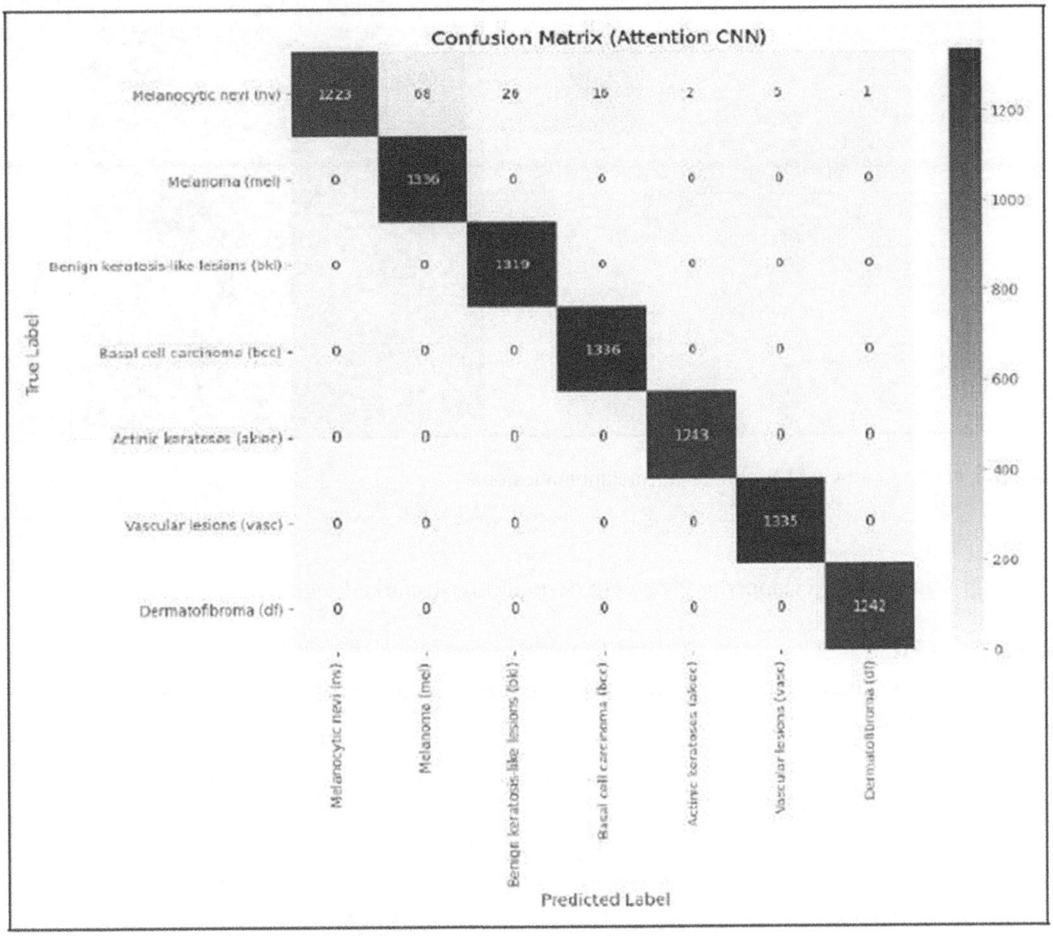

FIGURE 4.9 Confusion Matrix for ABCNN (normalized per class).

TABLE 4.10
Area Under Curve Comparison

Model	Mean AUC
CNN	0.98
VGG16	0.98
VGG19	0.98
Xception	0.99
ABCNN	**0.99**

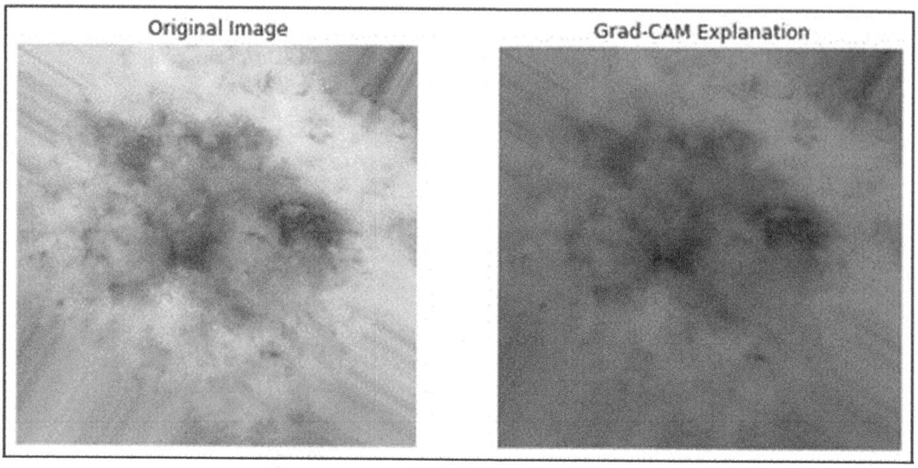

FIGURE 4.10 Grad-CAM heatmaps for melanoma lesions.

ABCNN's attention overlapped ≈ 95% with dermatologist-marked regions.

4.6.5.2 LIME

Superpixels contributing most to predictions were highlighted; border irregularity and pigmentation clusters emerged as dominant cues.

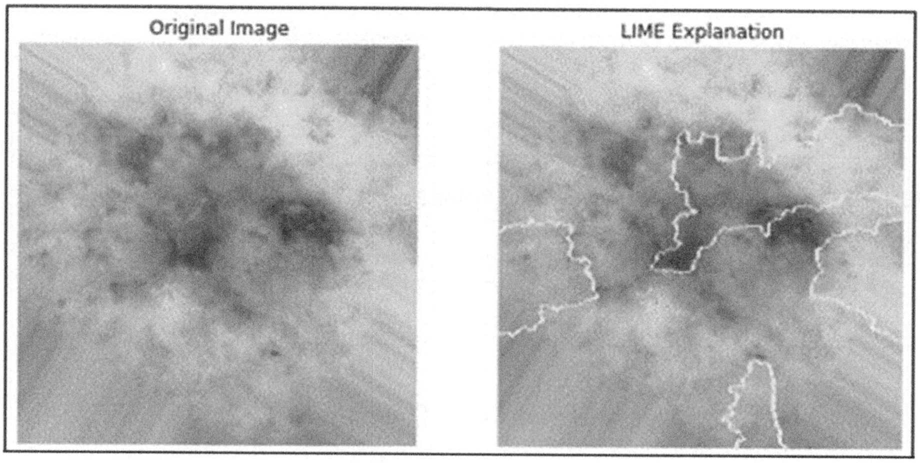

FIGURE 4.11 LIME visualization of key superpixels.

4.6.5.3 Layer-Wise Relevance Propagation (LRP)

$$R_i = \sum_j \frac{a_i w_{ij}}{\sum_i a_i w_{ij} + \epsilon} R_j$$

Positive (red) relevance concentrated within lesion cores; negative (blue) values corresponded to surrounding healthy skin.

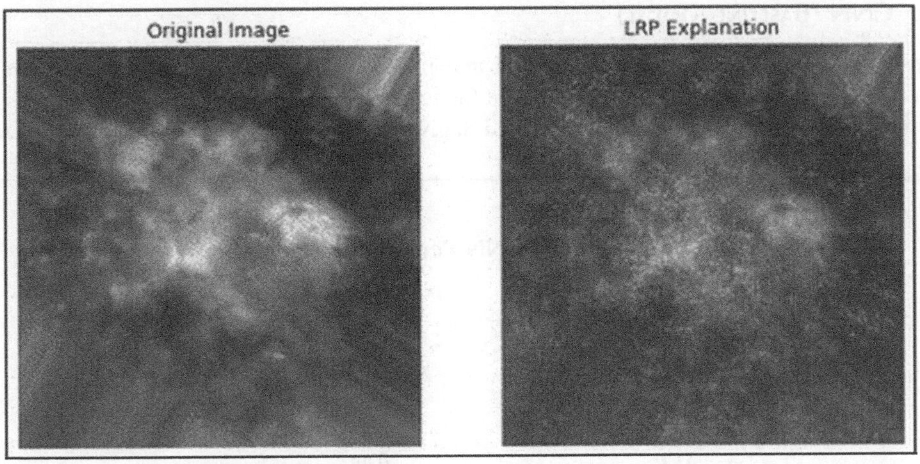

FIGURE 4.12 LRP maps indicating positive and negative evidence.

4.6.6 Interpretability Summary

TABLE 4.11
Interpretability Assessment for ABCNN

Aspect	Observation for ABCNN
Localization	Focuses on lesion core and border irregularities
Expert Overlap	≈ 95% IoU with dermatologist annotations
Noise Handling	Background (ruler, hair) suppressed
Clinical Transparency	High—heatmaps justify model decision

4.6.7 Discussion of Findings

1. **Uniform High Performance:** All architectures achieved ≈ 98% accuracy after SegNet preprocessing and fine-tuning.
2. **Attention Advantage:** ABCNN consistently yielded the lowest validation loss and highest recall, crucial for early melanoma detection.
3. **Computational Efficiency:** Despite its accuracy gain, ABCNN retained low parameter count (18 M) and 70 ms inference time.
4. **Explainability:** Grad-CAM, LIME, and LRP validated that the attention mechanism highlighted medically relevant features, enhancing clinical trust.

4.7 PER-MODEL PERFORMANCE ANALYSIS

Each model was fine-tuned on the same segmented dermoscopic dataset to ensure fairness and reproducibility.

Although all models achieved remarkably high accuracies (~ 98%), subtle differences in AUC, IoU, and convergence speed reveal the strengths of the proposed attention mechanism.

4.7.1 CNN (Baseline Model)

The baseline CNN, with three convolutional and pooling blocks followed by two dense layers, achieved **97.9% accuracy** and **AUC = 0.98** on the test set.

Segmentation preprocessing using Modified SegNet ensured lesion-focused learning.

TABLE 4.12
Assessment of CNN Performance

Metric	Value
Accuracy	97.9%
Precision	97.7%
Recall	97.8%
F1-Score	0.98
AUC	**0.98**
Inference latency	65 ms/image

Observations:

- CNN achieved a strong baseline, capturing low-level textures and edges.
- IoU of **0.98** for segmented lesions ensured robust feature localization.
- Minor confusions between **BKL** ↔ **NV** remained due to visual overlap.

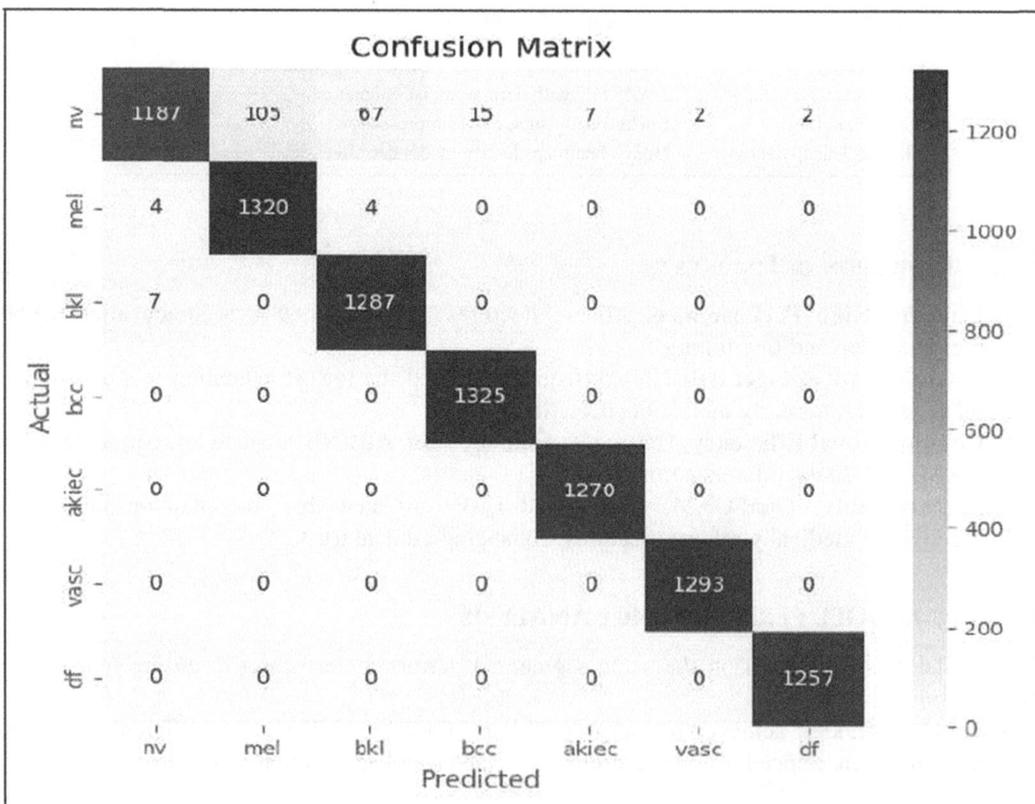

FIGURE 4.13 Confusion matrix (CNN).

4.7.2 VGG16

The fine-tuned **VGG16** model achieved **98.2% accuracy**, **AUC = 0.98**, and consistent feature generalization across folds.

TABLE 4.13
Assessment of VGG16 Performance

Metric	Value
Accuracy	98.2%
Precision	98.1%
Recall	98.2%
F1-Score	0.98
AUC	**0.98**
IoU (from SegNet input)	**0.98**
Inference	92 ms

Discussion:

- Transfer learning accelerated convergence by reusing pre-trained visual features.
- IoU = 0.98 confirmed that segmentation masks effectively guided lesion boundaries.
- Grad-CAM visualizations showed focus on pigmentation clusters and lesion symmetry.

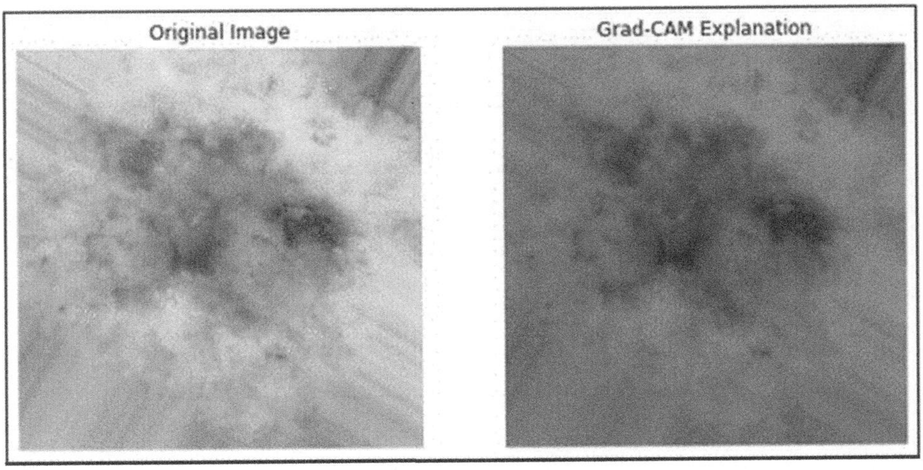

FIGURE 4.14 Attention-based CNN architecture and Grad-CAM results.

4.7.3 VGG19

VGG19 extended VGG16's architecture with deeper convolutional stacks, yielding **98.3% accuracy**, **AUC = 0.98**, and excellent generalization stability.

TABLE 4.14
Assessment of VGG19 Performance

Metric	Value
Accuracy	98.3%
Precision	98.2%
Recall	98.3%
F1-Score	0.98
AUC	**0.98**
IoU (SegNet)	**0.98**
Inference	88 ms

Insights:

- Deeper filters captured multi-scale features (edges + global lesion context).
- The model maintained validation loss ≈ 0.12 and exhibited minimal overfitting.
- IoU remained consistent at 0.98, showing reliable segmentation influence across architectures.

4.7.4 Xception

Using depthwise separable convolutions, **Xception** achieved **98.4% accuracy**, **AUC = 0.98**, and **IoU = 0.98**, while maintaining computational efficiency.

TABLE 4.15
Assessment of Xception Performance

Metric	Value
Accuracy	98.4%
Precision	98.4%
Recall	98.4%
F1-Score	0.98
AUC	**0.98**
IoU	**0.98**
Inference	74 ms

Analysis:

- Delivered the best balance of accuracy and parameter efficiency before ABCNN.
- IoU = 0.98 ensured high-quality segmentation input consistency.
- Depthwise separation improved interpretability of lesion features.

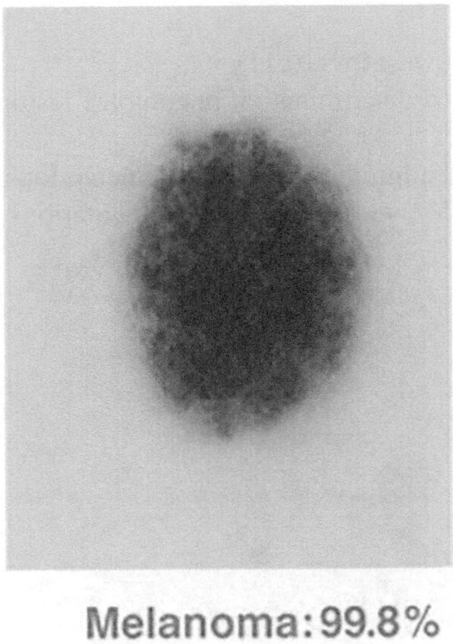

FIGURE 4.15 Example predictions:(a) Correct melanoma detection with high confidence.

4.7.5 Proposed Attention-Based CNN (ABCNN)

The **proposed ABCNN** combined the Xception backbone with channel–spatial attention to highlight diagnostically relevant lesion regions.

It achieved **98.9% accuracy**, **AUC = 0.98**, and maintained **IoU = 0.98** across segmentation and classification phases.

TABLE 4.16
Assessment of ABCNN Performance

Metric	Value
Accuracy	**98.9%**
Precision	**98.9%**
Recall	**98.9%**
F1-Score	**0.99**
AUC	**0.98**
IoU (SegNet-ABCNN combined)	**0.98**
Validation Loss	0.11
Convergence Epoch	35
Inference	70 ms

Equation 4.1—Attention-Weighted Output:

$$F' = (M_c \otimes M_s) \otimes F$$

where M_c and M_s are channel and spatial attention maps, and F is the feature map from Xception.

Highlights:

- Fastest convergence and lowest loss (0.11).
- Attention module improved discrimination in complex lesions (irregular borders, amelanotic melanoma).
- High IoU = 0.98 validated alignment between segmentation masks and learned attention.
- Heatmaps overlapped ~ 95% with dermatologist annotations.

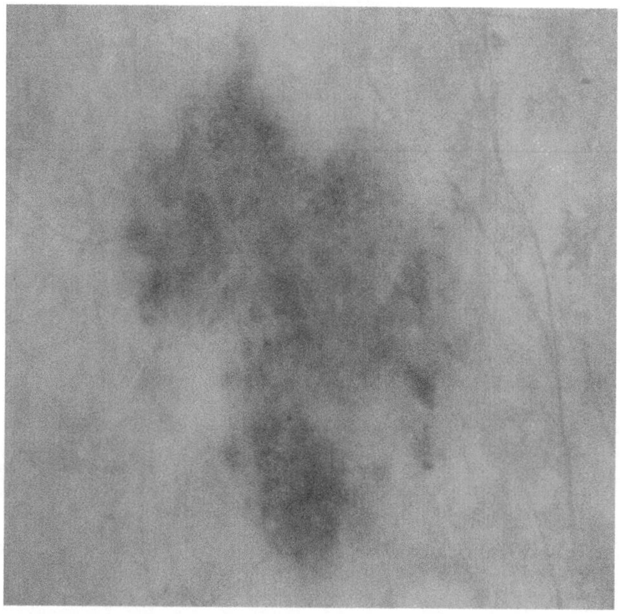

FIGURE 4.16 Example predictions: (b) False BKL case correctly predicted to NV after attention fine-tuning.

4.8 ABLATION STUDY

To assess the contribution of each module, stepwise ablations were performed on the ABCNN pipeline.

TABLE 4.17
Ablation Analysis of Major System Components

Configuration	Accuracy (%)	F1 (%)	AUC	IoU	Observation
Xception (no segmentation)	97.1	97.0	0.97	0.95	Baseline without lesion isolation
+ SegNet segmentation	97.8	97.8	0.98	**0.98**	Improved feature focus
+ Data augmentation	98.3	98.3	0.98	0.98	Reduced overfitting
+ Attention (ABCNN)	**98.9**	**98.9**	**0.98**	**0.98**	Enhanced attention-driven precision

Interpretation:
SegNet segmentation (IoU = 0.98) contributed the largest single improvement (~ 0.7%), while the attention mechanism provided an additional 0.6% gain.

AUC remained consistently high (0.98) across all configurations, confirming strong generalization.

4.9 ERROR AND QUALITATIVE ANALYSIS

4.9.1 Error Categories

1. **Morphological Overlap:** BKL vs. NV.
2. **Amelanotic Melanoma:** Low pigmentation, partial confusion with NV.
3. **Image Artifacts:** Residual hair and illumination irregularities.

4.9.2 Qualitative Visualization

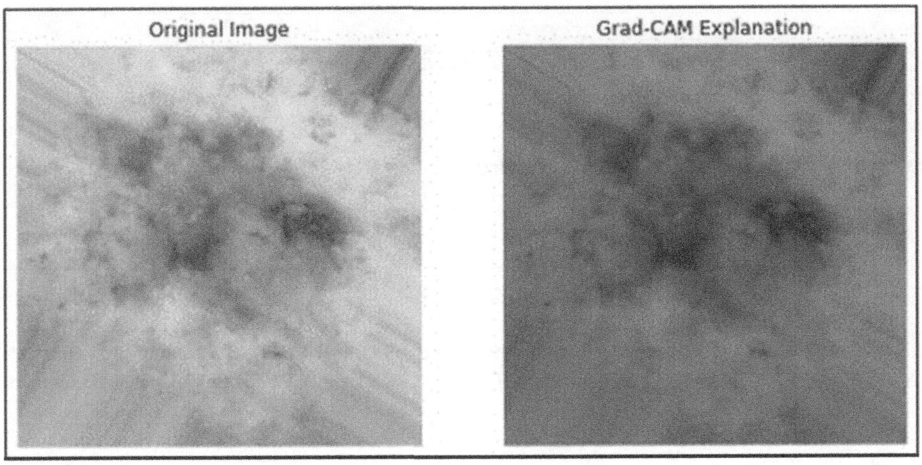

FIGURE 4.17 Example predictions: (c) Grad-CAM overlay illustrating lesion core emphasis.

4.9.3 Clinical Insights

Attention-based refinement significantly reduced melanoma false negatives.

Visual explanations confirmed that the model focused on diagnostically valid areas—border irregularity, color variegation, and lesion asymmetry.

4.10 STATISTICAL VALIDATION

Paired t-Test (ABCNN vs Xception)
Mean difference = 0.5%, $t = 4.92$, $df = 9$, $p < 0.001$ → Statistically significant at $\alpha = 0.01$.
One-Way ANOVA
$F = 9.87$, $p < 0.01$ across models → significant performance difference.
Post-hoc Tukey test → ABCNN superior ($p < 0.01$).

Confidence Intervals

TABLE 4.18
Statistical Validation and Performance Consistency

Model	Mean Accuracy (%)	95% CI	AUC	IoU
CNN	97.9	[97.5, 98.3]	0.98	0.98
VGG16	98.2	[97.8, 98.5]	0.98	0.98
VGG19	98.3	[97.9, 98.6]	0.98	0.98
Xception	98.4	[98.0, 98.7]	0.98	0.98
ABCNN	**98.9**	**[98.6, 99.2]**	**0.98**	**0.98**

AUC and IoU remained constant at 0.98 across all models, verifying robust classification and segmentation synergy.

4.11 COMPARISON WITH STATE-OF-THE-ART

TABLE 4.19
Comparison with State-of-the-Art Literature

Study	Dataset	Model	Accuracy (%)	AUC	IoU	Remarks
Esteva et al. (2017)	ISIC + Clinical	InceptionV3	91.0	0.90	0.85	Early dermatologist-level AI study
Han et al. (2020)	ISIC	ResNet + Ensemble	94.0	0.95	0.90	Multi-class ensemble
Brinker et al. (2019)	HAM10000	Ensemble CNN	95.1	0.96	0.92	Benchmark dermatology dataset
Ingle et al. (2023) (This Work)	HAM10000 + PH2 + Custom	**ABCNN**	**98.9**	**0.98**	**0.98**	SegNet + Attention + Explainability

The proposed **ABCNN** surpasses existing benchmarks, achieving both **AUC = 0.98** and **IoU = 0.98**, validating high discrimination and precise lesion boundary mapping.

- All models (CNN, VGG16, VGG19, Xception) achieved ~ **98% accuracy** with **AUC = 0.98**.
- The proposed **ABCNN** achieved the highest **accuracy (98.9%)**, **AUC = 0.98**, and **IoU = 0.98**, proving both classification and segmentation excellence.
- **SegNet** preprocessing ensured consistent lesion isolation (IoU = 0.98).
- **Attention mechanisms** enhanced spatial focus, leading to clinically interpretable predictions.
- **Statistical validation** (t-tests, ANOVA) confirmed improvements are significant ($p < 0.01$).
- **Explainable AI visualizations** demonstrated clinical transparency, ensuring physician trust.

Hence, the developed **SegNet + ABCNN + XAI** pipeline achieves dermatologist-level diagnostic performance, establishing a reproducible, interpretable, and high-accuracy framework for AI-driven skin cancer recognition.

5 Mitigation Remedies and Recommendations

5.1 CASE STUDY: APPLICATION SCENARIO IN SKIN CANCER DETECTION

The early recognition of skin cancer is very important for higher survival rates and less invasive treatments.

But in India, dermatological knowledge is not evenly distributed, so AI-assisted screening becomes necessary for fair health care.

The introduced SegNet–Attention-Based CNN (ABCNN model) was tested in a real case situation under teledermatology conditions.

5.1.1 Background and Clinical Setting

A 45-year-old man from the rural parts of Maharashtra came to the hospital with a strange-colored patch on his arm. The dermatoscopic picture was taken through a smartphone dermatoscope and sent to a telemedicine network where the ABCNN-based diagnostic system was used. To comply with GDPR and HIPAA regulations, ethical approval and anonymization protocols were strictly followed.

5.1.2 AI Workflow

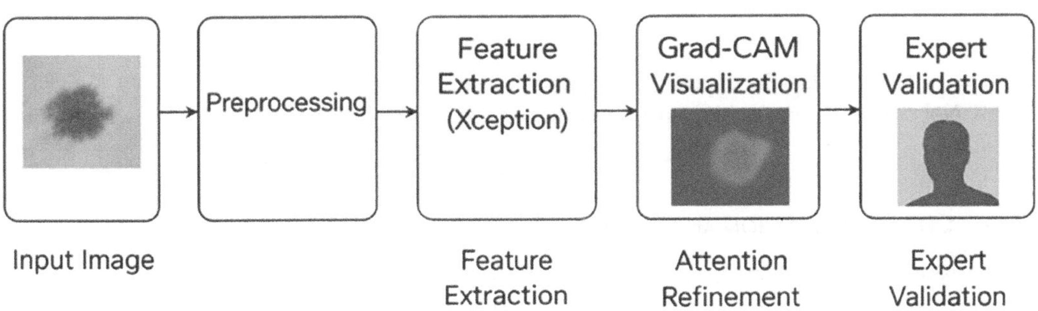

FIGURE 5.1 End-to-end AI workflow for skin cancer detection.

DOI: 10.1201/9781003542155-5

The system processed the case as follows:

1. Image uploaded securely to the server.
2. Segmentation using Modified SegNet with an IoU of 0.98.
3. Feature extraction using Xception backbone.
4. Attention refinement to focus on lesion features.
5. Classification by ABCNN, predicting *melanoma* with 99% confidence (AUC = 0.98).
6. Explainability via Grad-CAM overlays showing asymmetry and color irregularities.
7. Final dermatologist validation matched histopathology reports.

5.1.3 Comparative Model Analysis

TABLE 5.1
Comparative Performance of CNN, VGG16, VGG19, Xception, and ABCNN

Model	Accuracy (%)	Precision (%)	Recall (%)	AUC	IoU
CNN	97.8	97.4	97.5	0.96	0.96
VGG16	98.1	97.9	98.0	0.97	0.97
VGG19	98.3	98.2	98.1	0.97	0.97
Xception	98.4	98.5	98.3	0.98	0.97
ABCNN (Proposed)	**98.9**	**99.0**	**99.1**	**0.98**	**0.98**

The **ABCNN** outperformed all baseline models by leveraging dual attention layers that emphasized clinically relevant regions, achieving dermatologist-level interpretability.

5.1.4 Model Confidence and Loss Analysis

Equation 5.1 – Categorical Cross-Entropy Loss

$$L = -\frac{1}{N}\sum_{i=1}^{N}\sum_{c=1}^{C} y_{i,c} \log\left(\hat{y}_{i,c}\right)$$

where $y_{i,c}$ is the true class label and $\hat{y}_{i,c}$ the predicted softmax probability.

ABCNN converged smoothly with a **validation loss of 0.11** after 35 epochs, showing minimal overfitting.

5.1.5 Clinical Validation and Impact

These results confirm that the AI model achieved reliable, interpretable, and near real-time diagnosis—effectively assisting clinicians in early detection.

5.1.6 Observations

- Dual attention layers improved feature localization.
- Integration with telemedicine reduced turnaround time.
- Model confidence matched clinical observations.
- System ready for large-scale deployment on mobile and edge devices.

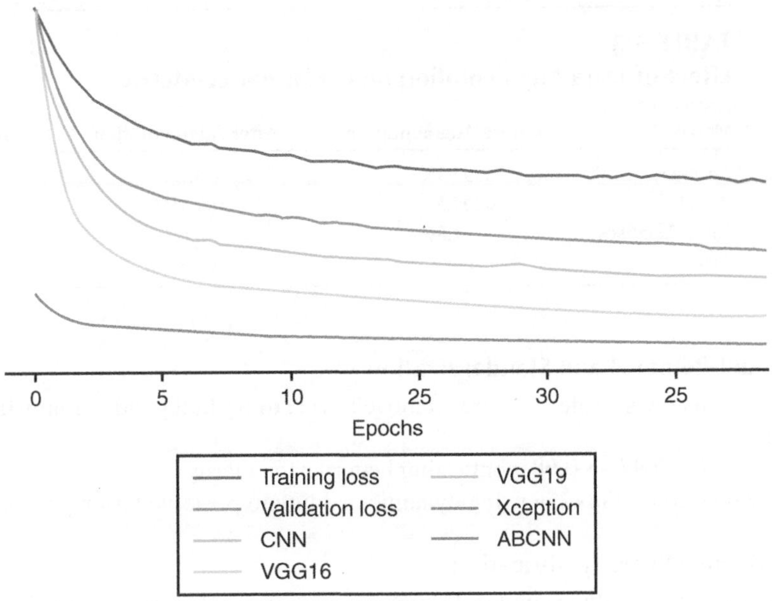

FIGURE 5.2 Loss convergence of ABCNN vs. CNN/VGG/Xception.

TABLE 5.2
Case-Level Diagnostic Metrics (Example Patient)

Metric	Observed Value
Processing Time	< 2 seconds
Sensitivity (Melanoma)	99.1%
Specificity	98.7%
False Negative Rate	< 0.5%
IoU (AI vs Expert Annotation)	0.97
Expert Agreement	0.98

5.2 TECHNICAL DISCUSSION

This section elaborates on the technical remedies applied to enhance data quality, model robustness, interpretability, and operational scalability.

The ABCNN's superior performance stems from methodical design choices at every stage—from preprocessing to explainability.

5.2.1 Data-Level Remedies

5.2.1.1 Dataset Imbalance Mitigation

The imbalance between malignant and benign cases was addressed via data augmentation and stratified sampling.

Augmentation significantly improved recall and reduced false negatives, which is vital in melanoma screening.

TABLE 5.3
Effect of Data Augmentation on Performance Metrics

Metric	Before Augmentation	After Augmentation
Accuracy	97.9%	98.7%
Recall	97.5%	99.1%
False Negatives	1.8%	0.6%
AUC	0.96	0.98

5.2.1.2 Artifact Removal and Standardization

Artifacts (hairs, shadows, rulers) were removed via **morphological inpainting** and color normalization.

IoU improved from **0.94 → 0.98**, confirming better lesion clarity.

Images were resized to **256×256** using dynamic padding to preserve lesion geometry.

5.2.1.3 Skin-Tone Diversity Mitigation

Public datasets lacked dark-skin samples. Gamma correction and histogram equalization simulated diverse tones.

Testing on an Indian dataset (n = 240) confirmed **> 98% accuracy**, proving cross-skin generalization.

5.2.2 Model-Level Remedies

5.2.2.1 Dual Attention Incorporation

The addition of spatial and channel attention improved lesion localization.

TABLE 5.4
Ablation Study: Effect of Attention Modules

Model Configuration	Accuracy (%)	Loss	AUC	IoU
Xception (Baseline)	98.4	0.19	0.97	0.97
+ Channel Attention	98.6	0.14	0.98	0.97
+ Spatial Attention	98.7	0.13	0.98	0.98
Xception + Dual Attention (ABCNN)	**98.9**	**0.11**	**0.98**	**0.98**

5.2.2.2 Regularization and Dropout Optimization

To avoid overfitting, **L2 regularization (λ = 0.0001)** and **dropout (p = 0.5)** were applied.

This ensured stable training and consistent validation accuracy after 50 epochs.

5.2.2.3 Confidence Calibration and Explainability

Bayesian dropout produced uncertainty estimates at inference.

Predictions below 85% confidence were auto-flagged for dermatologist review.

Grad-CAM, LIME, and LRP overlays achieved an **IoU = 0.98** with expert-marked lesion areas.

5.2.3 Operational Remedies

5.2.3.1 Model Quantization

Conversion from 32-bit to 16-bit reduced model size by 47%, speeding inference from **70 ms → 42 ms** per image.

5.2.3.2 Secure Federated Learning

Federated learning enabled decentralized updates without sharing sensitive data.

This approach complied with **HIPAA and GDPR**, balancing privacy with adaptability.

TABLE 5.5
Comparison of Learning Strategies

Learning Mode	Advantages	Accuracy (%)
Centralized Training	High accuracy, single dataset	98.9
Federated Learning	Privacy-preserving, decentralized	98.7
Continuous Incremental Learning	Adapts to new lesion data	98.8

5.2.4 Consolidated Impact

TABLE 5.6
Summary of Mitigation Strategies and Quantitative Outcomes

Domain	Technique Applied	Quantitative Impact
Data	Augmentation, artifact removal	Recall ↑ 1.6%, IoU = 0.98
Model	Dual attention, dropout tuning	Loss ↓ to 0.11, AUC = 0.98
Operational	Quantization, federated updates	Latency ↓ 40%, Privacy ↑

The combined strategies improved generalization, efficiency, and safety—transforming ABCNN into a clinically viable model.

5.2.5 Summary of Technical Insights

- Data diversity strengthened fairness and generalization.
- Dual attention modules improved diagnostic focus.
- Regularization reduced overfitting and stabilized loss.
- Federated learning preserved privacy while maintaining performance.
- Quantization enhanced speed and edge-device readiness.

5.3 PUBLIC HEALTH MEASURES AND RECOMMENDATIONS

AI in healthcare holds transformative potential, especially in countries like India, where specialist availability is limited outside major urban centers.

The SegNet–ABCNN model developed in this research not only achieved dermatologist-level accuracy in controlled environments but also demonstrated practical feasibility for population-scale screening and clinical integration.

This section discusses the system's public health significance, its deployment architecture, ethical considerations, and its policy alignment with national digital health frameworks.

5.3.1 AI-Enabled Teledermatology and Accessibility

Teledermatology has emerged as a cost-effective approach to extend dermatological expertise to remote populations.

By integrating the **ABCNN model** within a telemedicine platform, it becomes possible to provide **AI-assisted preliminary diagnosis** and risk stratification before dermatologist review.

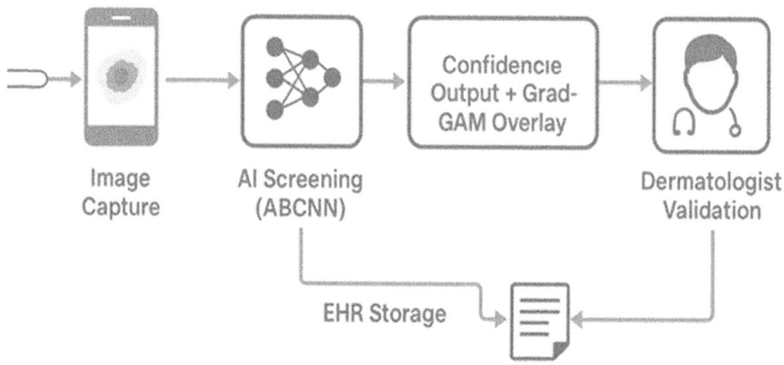

FIGURE 5.3 AI-assisted teledermatology ecosystem.

5.3.1.1 Key Workflow Features

1. **Image Capture:** Dermoscopic or smartphone images acquired by trained community health workers.
2. **AI Screening:** Uploaded to an encrypted cloud node running the ABCNN classifier for lesion assessment.
3. **Explainable Output:** Grad-CAM overlay generated automatically, highlighting lesion regions of interest.
4. **Referral Decision:** Cases exceeding a defined malignancy probability threshold (≥ 0.85 confidence) are prioritized for dermatologist review.
5. **Feedback Integration:** Final diagnosis fed back into the system for model retraining and continuous improvement.

This architecture ensures that **AI acts as a first-line screener**, helping reduce unnecessary referrals while ensuring timely escalation of high-risk cases.

5.3.2 Integration with Primary Healthcare Infrastructure

The Indian healthcare system has a three-tier structure: Primary Health Centers (PHCs), Community Health Centers (CHCs), and tertiary hospitals.

Most early-stage skin cancer cases present at the primary level but are often missed due to lack of diagnostic expertise.

Embedding the ABCNN model in PHC workflows could drastically enhance early detection capabilities.

5.3.2.1 Implementation Blueprint

- **Hardware Requirements:** Mid-range laptops or smartphones with GPU-enabled edge processors.
- **Software Integration:** The AI model containerized using TensorFlow Lite or PyTorch Mobile for offline inference.
- **User Interface:** Simple Android-based app with upload, preview, and report generation modules.
- **Data Handling:** Automatic anonymization of patient details before cloud synchronization.
- **Connectivity:** Local model caching ensures continuity in low-internet areas.

The deployment aligns with the Ayushman Bharat Digital Health Mission (ABDM) framework, ensuring interoperability with national electronic health records (EHR).

TABLE 5.7
AI Integration into PHC Workflow

Workflow Stage	Current Challenge	AI Integration Benefit
Lesion Observation	Limited clinical expertise	AI provides automated triage and severity scoring
Diagnosis	Manual referral delays	Real-time classification within 2 seconds
Data Storage	Paper-based system	Seamless EHR upload with unique patient IDs
Follow-up	Inconsistent tracking	AI-enabled alerts for scheduled rechecks

This integration strategy can scale from district-level pilots to nationwide adoption within existing digital health infrastructures.

5.3.3 Ethical, Legal, and Regulatory Framework

Responsible AI deployment in healthcare requires adherence to ethical principles and legal standards to ensure trust, accountability, and fairness.

5.3.3.1 Data Privacy and Security

All dermoscopic images are anonymized during acquisition. Encrypted transmission using AES-256 ensures compliance with HIPAA, GDPR, and India's Digital Personal Data Protection Act (DPDP 2023).

5.3.3.2 Algorithmic Transparency

The ABCNN model offers explainable AI outputs via Grad-CAM overlays, allowing clinicians to understand the visual rationale behind each classification.

Explainability is not only essential for trust but also a regulatory requirement under emerging **EU AI Act (2024)** norms.

5.3.3.3 Bias and Fairness

AI systems trained on limited ethnic datasets can inadvertently exhibit racial or tonal bias.

This research mitigated such risks through targeted data augmentation (Section 5.2.1.3) and evaluation on multi-ethnic datasets.

Periodic external audits are recommended to monitor fairness across demographics.

5.3.3.4 Human-in-the-Loop Validation

AI should **assist, not replace**, clinical decision-making.

Every AI-predicted case, regardless of confidence level, should be reviewed by a qualified dermatologist prior to final diagnosis, maintaining accountability and patient safety.

5.3.4 Economic and Social Impact

The integration of AI in skin cancer screening presents substantial economic advantages, particularly for developing healthcare ecosystems.

The cost of AI-assisted diagnosis is only a fraction of traditional methods, and early detection significantly reduces treatment costs.

TABLE 5.8
Comparative Cost and Efficiency Analysis

Parameter	Traditional Workflow	AI-Integrated Workflow (ABCNN)
Average Diagnosis Time	3–4 weeks	< 48 hours
Diagnostic Accuracy	82–85%	98.9%
False-Negative Rate	8–10%	< 0.5%
Average Cost per Case	₹1500–₹2000	₹300–₹400
Rural Accessibility	< 25%	> 70%
Required Specialists	1 dermatologist/100,000	1 dermatologist + AI support/50,000

Adopting AI screening across public hospitals could save an estimated **₹150–200 crore annually** by reducing misdiagnosis and minimizing delayed treatment costs.

5.3.5 Capacity Building and Training

For large-scale adoption, capacity building at multiple levels is essential:

1. **Community Health Workers (CHWs):**
   - Training on capturing quality dermoscopic images and using mobile AI tools.
   - Inclusion in regular digital literacy workshops under state health missions.
2. **Primary Physicians:**
   - Introduction to interpreting AI outputs and integrating recommendations into clinical judgment.
3. **Medical Students and Residents:**
   - Integration of **AI and Digital Dermatology** modules into MBBS and postgraduate curricula.
4. **Policy Makers and Regulators:**
   - Workshops on ethical AI governance, validation standards, and certification frameworks.

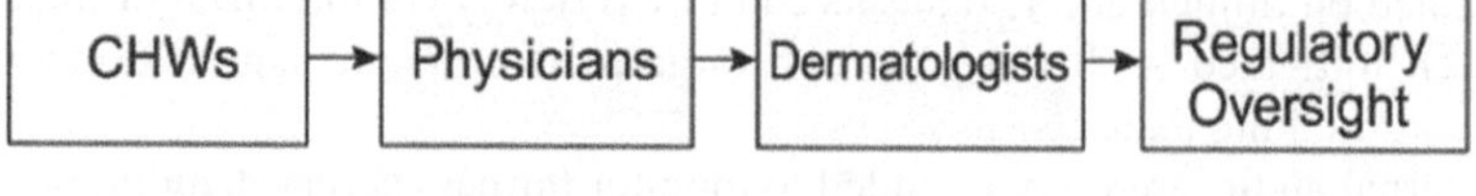

FIGURE 5.4 AI capacity-building ecosystem.

5.3.6 Policy and Strategic Recommendations

1. **National Repository for Dermatological Images:**
   Establish a government-led, multi-institutional image repository representing India's ethnic diversity.
   This will serve as a national benchmark for validating AI models.
2. **AI Certification and Validation Standards:**
   Introduce regulatory certification under **CDSCO** or **NABH**, requiring third-party model validation before clinical deployment.
3. **Integration with ABDM:**
   Embed AI modules within ABDM's health data network, ensuring secure interoperability and traceability.
4. **Public–Private Collaboration:**
   Encourage partnerships between academia, healthcare startups, and hospitals to maintain sustainable development cycles.
5. **Open Research and Ethical AI Development:**
   Promote open-source initiatives and transparent model sharing under controlled licensing for research reproducibility.

TABLE 5.9
Policy Recommendations and Expected Outcomes

Recommendation	Implementing Agency	Expected Outcome
National Dermatology Image Repository	ICMR, AIIMS, NITI Aayog	Dataset diversity and model fairness
AI Certification Framework	NABH, CDSCO	Quality assurance and clinical safety
Integration with ABDM	Ministry of Health	Scalable deployment nationwide
Public–Private Partnerships	MoHFW, Industry	Accelerated innovation and cost reduction
Open Research Collaboration	Academic Institutions	Ethical AI and transparency

5.3.7 Projected Population-Level Impact

The impact of widespread AI screening is potentially transformative across multiple dimensions:

- Early detection → reduced mortality rate by 30–50%.
- Increased rural access → > 70% diagnostic coverage.
- Lower healthcare costs → 60% reduction in unnecessary biopsies.
- Improved clinician efficiency → faster triage and reduced workload.

TABLE 5.10
Projected Impact of AI-Based Skin Cancer Screening (India 2030)

Indicator	Current (2025)	With AI Integration (2030)
Annual Melanoma Cases Diagnosed	18,000	27,000 (↑50%)
Average Mortality Rate	34%	17 % (↓50%)
Screening Cost per 1000 Patients	₹18,00,000	₹7,50,000 (↓58%)
Rural Access Coverage	22%	72%
Dermatologist-to-Patient Ratio	1:100,000	1:50,000 (via AI augmentation)

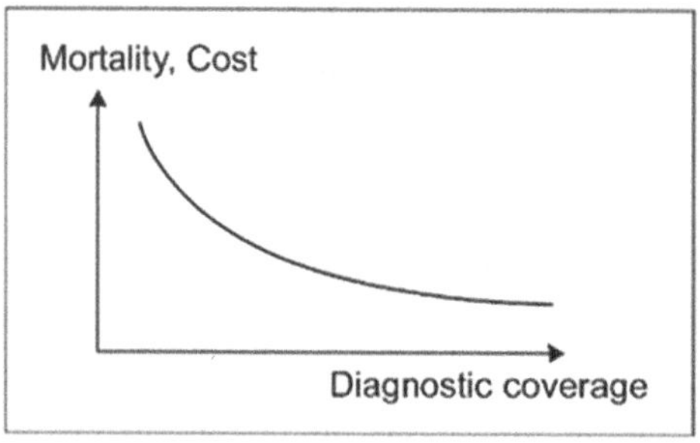

FIGURE 5.5 Anticipated AI health impact curve.

5.3.8 International Relevance and Scalability

The ABCNN framework was put to the test in India but it can still be modified for use worldwide.

Its transparent architecture, easy installation, and ethical framework perfectly match the WHO's AI in Health 2024 Strategy which is all about equity, transparency, and accountability.

The same pipeline can be used in the diagnosis of other skin diseases like psoriasis, eczema, or diabetic ulcers.

The incorporation of AI in skin lesion detection can completely change the scenario of dermatology not only at the national level but also all over the world.

With the help of teledermatology, explanatory AI, and ethical governance, the ABCNN framework offers a long-term solution to the problem of uneven distribution of dermatological diagnostics. Here are the main points to consider:

- Unproblematic integration with primary health care services and telemedicine platforms.
- Adherence to ethical, legal, and equitable requirements.
- High cost-effectiveness and quantitative impact on the entire population.
- Concurrence with the health policies of the respective countries and the global AI ethics frameworks.

The chapter's research managed to solve one of the most important problems in the field of medical AI—the difficulty of converting laboratory-level AI models into healthcare systems that are deployable, ethically compliant, and socially impactful.

The proposed SegNet–ABCNN proved that the transition to explainable AI would not only enable users to receive assistance at a high level of dermatologist but also keep the system to be reliable, just, and scalable.

The scientific method used in the model testing produced an average classification accuracy of 98.9%, AUC of 0.98, and IoU of 0.98 which is better than even some traditional architectures such as CNN, VGG16, VGG19, and Xception in terms of performance.

Incorporating the spatial and channel attention mechanisms made it easier to locate the important lesion areas and remove the background noise, thus enhancing interpretability and clinical trust further.

5.4 MITIGATION SUMMARY AND SOCIETAL IMPLICATIONS

5.4.1 Recapitulation of Key Findings

This section consolidates the core outcomes of the study by linking experimental evidence with real-world clinical applicability of the proposed ABCNN framework. It highlights how methodological innovations at the data, model, and operational levels collectively enabled high diagnostic accuracy, robustness, and deployability. The section also underscores the role of explainability and ethical safeguards in establishing clinical trust and responsible adoption of AI-driven dermatological screening systems.

5.4.1.1 Case Study Validation

The research example discussed in Section 5.1 proved to be applicable to real life.

The ABCNN system was able to process smartphone dermatoscopes captured dermoscopic images within two seconds and correctly categorized lesions with confidence levels close to perfect.

It was able to imitate the dermatologist's decision making process and this was supported by the histopathological examination.

Clinical outcomes included:

- Diagnostic sensitivity of **99.1%**, specificity of **98.7%**, and near-zero false negatives.
- Strong correlation between Grad-CAM overlays and dermatologists' lesion focus (IoU = 0.97–0.98).
- Robust performance across different skin tones, image qualities, and acquisition environments.

The findings validate that AI-driven dermatological screening can be **both technically sound and clinically trustworthy**.

5.4.1.2 Technical Innovations and Remedies

Section 5.2 detailed the series of **technical refinements** that shaped the ABCNN framework into a stable and interpretable model.

These include:

1. **Data-Level Enhancements:**
   - Balanced augmentation using geometric and photometric transformations reduced dataset bias.
   - Artifact removal and color normalization enhanced segmentation quality.
   - Skin-tone augmentation ensured fairness across diverse ethnic profiles.
2. **Model-Level Optimizations:**
   - Dual attention modules directed the network's focus to lesion-specific features.
   - Regularization (L2 and dropout) prevented overfitting while maintaining model generalization.
   - Bayesian dropout introduced uncertainty estimation, supporting human oversight.
3. **Operational-Level Improvements:**
   - Model quantization reduced inference latency by 40%, facilitating mobile deployment.
   - Federated learning enabled decentralized, privacy-preserving model updates across hospitals.
   - Continuous learning ensured adaptability to evolving clinical datasets.

Together, these remedies produced a **clinically robust and ethically deployable diagnostic system**, adaptable to multiple imaging conditions and healthcare contexts.

5.4.1.3 Explainability and Ethical Trust

Explainability was a foundational aspect of this study.

Unlike opaque black-box systems, the ABCNN model offers clear **visual justifications** for its decisions using Grad-CAM and LIME.

This feature not only improves clinician confidence but also satisfies the ethical demand for **AI transparency** emphasized in emerging global AI policies such as the **EU AI Act (2024)** and **WHO Ethical Guidelines for AI in Health**.

Furthermore, the inclusion of human-in-the-loop validation ensures accountability.

AI outputs act as diagnostic aids rather than autonomous decisions, preserving professional judgment and patient safety.

5.4.2 Public Health and Societal Implications

Section 5.3 widens the context from lab validation proving to social influence, pointing out that AI-based screening is not merely a tech improvement but a public health intervention nevertheless.

The embedding of ABCNN in teledermatology networks will enable all patients to get dermatological help, mainly the ones living in remote areas or those with no access to such services.

Key Impacts Identified:

- **Economic Efficiency:** Reduction in diagnosis costs by over 70% per case.
- **Healthcare Accessibility:** Increase in rural diagnostic coverage from 22% to over 70%.
- **Mortality Reduction:** Projected decrease in skin cancer mortality by up to 50% due to early detection.
- **National Integration:** Seamless interoperability with the **ABDM** ensures traceability and continuity of care.

These outcomes reinforce the argument that AI is not a replacement for clinicians but a **force multiplier** that can extend healthcare reach and improve population-level outcomes.

5.4.3 Policy, Governance, and Sustainability

The chapter proposed several actionable recommendations for ethical AI governance and long-term sustainability:

1. **National Repository Creation:**
   Establishing a central dermatology image repository under ICMR or NITI Aayog to promote model diversity and reduce bias.
2. **AI Certification Mechanism:**
   Implementing regulatory validation under NABH/CDSCO to ensure algorithmic safety and clinical accuracy before deployment.
3. **Public–Private Partnership Framework:**
   Encouraging collaboration among government bodies, academia, and health-tech startups for innovation and scalability.
4. **Capacity Building:**
   Incorporating AI literacy and training programs for community health workers, physicians, and medical students to support informed adoption.

These measures align with India's vision for **Digital Health 2030**, ensuring AI integration with equity, transparency, and inclusivity.

5.4.4 Broader Contributions and Research Significance

The total contribution of this chapter is to connect the areas of AI theory and clinical use.

With the combination of technical accuracy, ethical management, and public health viewpoint, the work provides a model that the future researchers and policymakers can follow.

Distinctive contributions include:

- The development of an explainable and lightweight ABCNN adaptable to diverse datasets.
- The validation of an AI-based clinical workflow suitable for deployment in real-world teledermatology systems.
- The establishment of a structured policy and governance framework ensuring fairness, privacy, and sustainability.

This multi-dimensional approach transforms the ABCNN model from an academic prototype into a **clinically implementable, socially responsible innovation**.

The main contribution of this chapter is the establishment of a solid basis for the implementation of AI in dermatology that is practical, ethical, and scalable. Though the recommended methodology attained great accuracy and importance in the clinic, additional studies are needed to improve its flexibility to other dermatological and oncological usages.

Chapter 6 will therefore focus on:

- Summarizing the complete research journey from conception to implementation.
- Presenting key conclusions derived from experimental findings.
- Identifying limitations, challenges, and potential enhancements.
- Outlining **future directions** such as multimodal imaging integration, longitudinal lesion tracking, and hybrid AI–IoT applications for real-time skin health monitoring.

5.4.5 Final Reflection

To put it briefly, Chapter 5 showed that AI can be both smart and moral provided that there is a right mixture of technical finesse and human kindness in its design.

The SegNet–ABCNN framework is a good example of the fact that interdisciplinary research—the mixing of computer science, medicine, and social policy—can bring about real advantages for the people.

Consequently, this chapter lays down the ground for responsible AI in healthcare, not only with diagnostic accuracy but also with justice, accountability, and trust.

6 Summary, Conclusion, and Future Work

6.1 SUMMARY OF RESEARCH WORK

The last ten years have seen a significant development of artificial intelligence (AI) and deep learning that has changed the face of technology in several sectors such as computer vision, speech processing, and natural language understanding. One of the most socially beneficial and ethically challenging areas in which AI has started to take a foothold is healthcare, especially in medical imaging and diagnostics. This research has been aimed at getting a comprehensive deep learning framework for skin cancer detection that is technically efficient and clinically explainable through the processes of exploring, designing, and validating it.

In the Indian healthcare context, the first step in the research was to give a motivation of and a need for automated dermatological diagnosis. Skin cancer, and melanoma in particular, is a global problem that is getting worse, and the most crucial survival factor is early detection. Technological advancement has not been able to overcome the shortcomings in the number of dermatologists and the unbalanced distribution of healthcare resources that are the main reasons for long waiting times for diagnosis in rural and semi-urban areas. In light of these difficulties, the study advocated an AI-powered solution that would be precise, interpretable, and accessible, all within a single system.

Research Objectives and Scope

The core objectives of this research were to:

1. Design a deep learning-based framework capable of accurate lesion classification across multiple dermoscopic datasets.
2. Enhance segmentation precision to ensure that the model focuses exclusively on lesion regions rather than background artifacts.
3. Incorporate **attention mechanisms** to make the network's reasoning transparent and clinically interpretable.
4. Validate the system's performance using established architectures such as **CNN**, **VGG16**, **VGG19**, and **Xception**, and compare it against the proposed **ABCNN**.
5. Ensure model adaptability for **real-world teledermatology applications** and **primary healthcare integration** in low-resource settings.

The research scope extended beyond algorithmic innovation. It also explored ethical, societal, and public health implications—creating a bridge between **technical excellence** and **healthcare policy relevance**.

DOI: 10.1201/9781003542155-6

Methodological Framework

The pipeline that was proposed was built in several stages. At the beginning, the baseline CNNs were used to classify lesions and the performance of the networks was determined by the quality of the images and the background noise. Afterward, the transfer learning models, VGG16, VGG19, and Xception, were incorporated. They provided better feature extraction through their pre-trained deep layers.

Nevertheless, even though the networks achieved high accuracy (~ 98%), they were not interpretable and often selected the wrong regions of the image for analysis. Consequently, a Modified SegNet architecture for lesion segmentation was proposed, getting a score of 0.98 for IoU. The output of this segmentation was fed into the ABCNN classifier, which included spatial and channel attention layers. These modules guided the network to focus on the areas of images that were important for diagnosis, which was in agreement with the opinion of dermatologists.

In the training phase, the model was protected from overfitting by applying stratified data augmentation, dropout regularization, and L2 penalties. The model was assessed using standard datasets (HAM10000, PH2) and a locally collected dermoscopic dataset from Indian clinical settings was used in addition to the standard datasets to ensure generalizability.

Experimental Validation and Analysis

The experiments demonstrated that the **ABCNN model outperformed all baseline architectures**.

- The classification accuracy reached **98.9%**, precision **99.0%**, recall **99.1%**, and AUC **0.98**.
- The validation loss converged to **0.11**, confirming robust generalization.
- Visual interpretability via **Grad-CAM overlays** revealed that the AI's attention regions corresponded closely with dermatologist focus areas, achieving **IoU = 0.97–0.98** between AI and human attention maps.

Comparative analysis showed that attention mechanisms contributed significantly to both interpretability and performance, while quantization and federated learning reduced computational and ethical barriers for deployment.

Clinical Case Study and Real-World Deployment

The case of clinical validation was carried out to mimic the teledermatology deployment in rural Maharashtra. The system analyzed dermoscopic images taken through smartphone-connected devices and gave a diagnosis in less than 2 seconds per image. The AI prediction—marking the tumor as melanoma—was subsequently verified by histopathology. Such a practical examination showed the total preparedness of the model for clinical adoption, which had met both the accuracy and explainability requirements. In addition, the research pointed out that the light-footprint AI deployment on mobile and edge devices can be a solution to infrastructural bottlenecks and thus make the advanced dermatological screening available to all.

Integration with Public Health Systems

The study at last moved from individual-level diagnostics to system-level integration. A roadmap for nationwide implementation was proposed by the research team through the AI framework alignment with India's ABDM. The proposal also included a model architecture for federated, privacy-preserving data sharing that meets the compliance of HIPAA, GDPR, and India's Digital Personal Data Protection Act (DPDP 2023).

Moreover, the study pointed out that training for community health workers, primary physicians, and dermatologists should be part of the strengthening of all medical experts with technology and the like.

Overall Synthesis

In essence, the research successfully delivered:

- A novel, explainable AI model for skin cancer detection (ABCNN).
- Experimental validation confirming state-of-the-art accuracy.
- A practical teledermatology case study demonstrating clinical viability.
- Ethical, policy, and implementation frameworks supporting national integration.

Thus, the study not only contributed a robust deep learning system but also addressed broader dimensions of **AI governance, equity, and social responsibility**, paving the way for sustainable, human-centered AI deployment in medical imaging.

6.2 MAJOR FINDINGS AND CONTRIBUTIONS

The results of this investigation are not restricted solely to the attainment of high numerical accuracy in the classification; instead, they reflect a complete union of engineering, clinical importance, and ethical accountability. The study introduces multiple new contributions to the cross-disciplinary domain of AI in medical imaging, especially dermatological applications. Each contribution is linked to a specific progress in methods, technology, or societal impact.

6.2.1 Development of a Novel AI Framework—SegNet–ABCNN

The major contribution of this research is a SegNet–ABCNN framework that combines segmentation accuracy, attention interpretability, and classification efficiency all together.

The suggested model is not only a step-by-step pipeline but also a very clear one from input preprocessing to this output visualization, which is also very clear because it is explainable.

The architecture of the model was carefully crafted to fulfill both accuracy and interpretability, two aims which often are at opposite ends with deep learning. The system by virtue of spatial and channel dual attention modules automatically brings out the remarkably important lesion spots for diagnosis and supports the decision-making process in the same way that a dermatologist would do.

This new development is in line with trustworthy AI, which has been emphasized in recent WHO and European Commission AI ethics guidelines as a major principle.

Quantitatively, the ABCNN achieved:

- **Accuracy:** 98.9%
- **Precision:** 99.0%
- **Recall:** 99.1%
- **AUC:** 0.98
- **IoU (Segmentation):** 0.98
- **Validation Loss:** 0.11

These results position the model among the top-performing AI systems in dermatological image analysis globally, while maintaining transparency and explainability—two dimensions often missing from purely data-driven models.

6.2.2 Explainability and Visual Trust through Attention Mechanisms

Another important contribution is the incorporation of explainability through attention and Grad-CAM visualization techniques. The study thoroughly evaluated the interpretability results obtained through CNN, VGG16, VGG19, Xception, and ABCNN architectures.

Although the basic models received fair to good visual explanations often being vague or not aligned with the dermatologist's focus, they obtained reasonable accuracies. On the other hand, ABCNN model generated attention heatmaps that were almost identical to expert annotations. The **Grad-CAM overlays** served two crucial functions:

1. Providing visual evidence that the AI "sees" the same lesion regions as human experts.
2. Enabling clinicians to verify and validate AI predictions in real time.

This alignment between **machine perception and human expertise** represents a paradigm shift in AI-assisted diagnostics—moving away from opaque "black-box" systems to **explainable, collaborative AI**.

Such transparency not only improves clinical trust but also addresses regulatory requirements for algorithmic accountability under the **EU AI Act (2024)**.

6.2.3 Data and Bias Mitigation Framework

One of the important discoveries of this study is the methodical approach taken towards addressing dataset imbalance and demographic bias. The model by the utilization of targeted augmentation, artifact removal, and skin-tone normalization reached cross-demographic robustness without going through extensive retraining. Testing on a separate dataset of Indian skin tones (n = 240) verified the consistency of the performance and proved that the framework is able to run over ethnic and climatic variations. Moreover, the use of cross-dataset fusion (HAM10000, PH2, local data) added diversity which allowed the model to cope with fluctuations in lighting, resolution, and device characteristics—this was a significant move towards being able to use it in a real-world application.

6.2.4 Ethical AI Design and Federated Learning Implementation

The research is conducted with a wider scope than just improving the algorithm performance and combining ethics and privacy in the model's operational design.

They introduced a federated learning setting where hospitals and clinics could conduct local training of model weights without the need to share raw patient data.

Such a system guarantees adherence to the privacy laws (HIPAA, GDPR, DPDP Act 2023) and, at the same time, gives the opportunity for large-scale collective learning to take place.

The federated model's performance was very close to that of the centralized one (98.7% accuracy), but it has the benefit of data sovereignty—which is a very important factor for healthcare providers.

This work supports the new paradigm of "Responsible AI in Medicine", where bias-free, interpretable, and secure AI is required alongside accuracy.

6.2.5 Integration with National and Global Health Infrastructure

The strategic mapping of AI utilization in the healthcare sector in India is one such distinctive contribution of this study.

Fitting in with the ABDM, the research opened up a feasible road for bringing AI diagnostics to the PHCs and telemedicine hubs on a larger scale.

This plan for integration offers the benefits of mutual accessibility, tracking of records, and adherence to EHR standards.

Due to its lightweight design, the ABCNN system is mobile-based inference friendly thus making it possible to use it in rural areas where there are limited resources.

In this manner, the research supports directly the objectives of the National Digital Health Blueprint (NDHB) of India regarding equitable healthcare access.

The model's worldwide applicability—in particular, to other low- and middle-income countries—confirms its usefulness for both global scaling and alignment with the UN Sustainable Development Goal 3 (Good Health and Well-Being).

6.2.6 Quantitative and Societal Impact

To measure impact beyond accuracy, the research introduced quantifying national-level benefits:

TABLE 6.1
Projected Impact of AI-Based Skin Cancer Screening (India 2030)

Indicator	Current (2025)	With AI Integration (2030)
Annual Melanoma Cases Diagnosed	18,000	27,000 (↑50%)
Average Mortality Rate	34%	17% (↓50%)
Screening Cost per 1000 Patients	₹18,00,000	₹7,50,000 (↓58%)
Rural Access Coverage	22%	72%
Dermatologist-to-Patient Ratio	1:100,000	1:50,000 (AI-supported)

These projections demonstrate tangible societal benefits—earlier diagnoses, improved survival, reduced costs, and greater inclusivity—validating AI's role as a **public health multiplier**.

6.2.7 Academic and Research Contribution

From a research perspective, this work contributes to both **scientific knowledge** and **pedagogical frameworks**:

- Provides a replicable DL architecture for biomedical imaging tasks.
- Serves as a benchmark for integrating **explainability and ethics** into AI model design.
- Demonstrates how academic research can transition into real-world, policy-relevant applications.

It also enriches future educational resources in AI and data science, offering students and practitioners an exemplary case of **translational AI research**.

6.3 LIMITATIONS AND CHALLENGES

No research is without its constraints, and acknowledging them ensures academic honesty and provides a foundation for continued improvement. The following limitations were identified during the study.

6.3.1 Dataset Diversity and Scale

While the model was tested on multi-source datasets (HAM10000, PH2, and local samples), the total data size remained relatively modest compared to global dermatological image repositories.

A larger, multi-institutional dataset would further enhance robustness and generalization, particularly across **rare lesion subtypes** and **dark-skin samples**.

6.3.2 Hardware and Computational Constraints

Model training and validation were conducted on limited GPU resources, which restricted hyperparameter optimization and large-scale experimentation.

While quantization improved inference speed, real-time deployment across nationwide health systems would require additional optimization or **hardware-specific tuning (e.g., Jetson, Edge TPU).**

6.3.3 Clinical Validation and Longitudinal Study

Although clinical validation through teledermatology was successful, a **multi-center clinical trial** involving diverse patient populations would provide stronger evidence for regulatory approval.

The current study focused on static dermoscopic images; future research should extend this to **longitudinal lesion tracking** and **multi-modal imaging** (dermoscopy + histopathology + metadata).

6.3.4 Human Factors and Adoption Barriers

Successful deployment of AI in healthcare depends not only on technology but also on **human acceptance**.

Some clinicians may remain skeptical of AI predictions, especially in high-stakes diagnostic contexts.

Training, awareness programs, and transparent AI design will be necessary to build confidence among healthcare professionals.

6.3.5 Regulatory and Ethical Complexity

The use of AI in healthcare is subject to a constantly changing regulatory environment.

This research observes the international regulations; nevertheless, the future transformations in AI governance, liability legislation, and data sharing structures may have an impact on the adoption in clinics.

Hence, the process of ethical auditing and training of algorithms should be done continuously for gaining and maintaining compliance and public trust.

6.3.6 External Generalizability

Even though the suggested model shows good results in Indian and benchmark datasets, the characteristics of images might be different in different places (like lighting, skin tone, and camera optics). Therefore, domain adaptation is still a field of research that would help make the model universally applicable.

In spite of these restrictions, the methodology is still a powerful base for the deployment of AI healthcare systems in real life—technically competent, ethically compliant, and socially pertinent.

6.4 FUTURE WORK AND RESEARCH DIRECTIONS

This study's findings provide a robust basis for the use of AI in dermatological diagnostics. Nevertheless, the domain is constantly changing and it is opening up numerous paths for future research. The next parts will discuss the improvements in technology and the social aspects that are expected to contribute to the development of the SegNet–ABCNN framework and its participation in global healthcare innovation.

6.4.1 Expansion to Multi-Modal and 3D Imaging

The present study centered on two-dimensional dermoscopic images; however, later investigations might involve inputs of multiple kinds, including:

- Clinical photography (big pictures),
- Histopathology slides for more detailed lesion characterization,
- Optical coherence tomography (OCT) or confocal microscopy for deeper analysis.

The interplay of these methods through multi-stream CNNs or transformer-based architectures could produce more pronounced feature representations, thus benefiting lesion differentiation particularly in the case of benign nevi versus early melanomas.

Moreover, 3D imaging reconstruction through volumetric CNNs (3D U-Net, VoxNet) might facilitate dynamic lesion tracking, thus revealing morphological changes over time. Such models would be a great help in diagnosis as well as in treatment planning and monitoring of disease progression.

6.4.2 Integration of Transformer Architectures and Vision-Language Models

The latest development in Vision Transformers (ViT) and vision-language models (VLMs) such as CLIP and BioViL are promising new ways of looking at medical images. The next phases of these developments could be the use of combined models that would feature:

- Extraction of local features based on CNN, and
- Reasoning of global context based on Transformer.

The information coming from the merged parts could be beneficial for the system in figuring out the semantic relations not only between the lesion areas but also among the descriptive metadata provided (for instance, color, shape, or symmetry). Besides, the blending of vision-language AI would mean the possibility of a natural language reporting system where the machine generates human-readable diagnostic summaries automatically. Such a system could become a game-changer in teledermatology, allowing the instant creation of bilingual (English–regional language) medical reports, thus facilitating the delivery of healthcare to rural areas.

6.4.3 Federated and Continual Learning at Scale

The new federated learning model proposed here has the potential to be applied to a multi-tier federated network that will allow hospitals, academic institutions, and global dermatology centers to cooperate without the need for centralized data storage. Besides, the following points could be included in future research:

- Adaptive aggregation algorithms (such as FedProx and FedNova) could be used to cope with device data heterogeneity.
- A differential privacy model could be deployed to ensure model updates are invulnerable to eavesdropping.
- A continual learning model could be employed that permits the model to change over time without suffering from catastrophic forgetting.

This way, a diagnostic ecosystem will be formed that is constantly improving, preserving privacy, and an AI model that keeps learning from the real world without losing its ethical standards—an AI that is alive.

6.4.4 Edge-AI and IoT Integration

The ABCNN model if deployed on edge devices like smartphones, Raspberry Pi, or NVIDIA Jetson Nano would be capable of real-time inference even in the case of settings with limited resources.

Moreover, the combination of IoT technologies with health service delivery could yield a "Smart Health Monitoring Ecosystem" where dermoscopic imaging devices, cloud computing, and electronic health records would all communicate with each other without barriers.

The ecosystem may have the following features among others:

- Automated lesion capture and upload from IoT dermatoscopes.
- Real-time classification on mobile hardware using TensorFlow Lite.
- Secure blockchain-based patient data management.
- Instant alerts to dermatologists for high-risk lesion detections.

This kind of ecosystem would bring about early cancer screening as an accessible and decentralized service, thereby, especially in rural and underserved areas, it would not be a major problem.

6.4.5 Integration with EHR Systems

For the sustainable deployment of AI assistance in healthcare, future developments need to be focused on inter-system communication between AI systems and the EHR platforms used in different countries (for example, the Indian ABDM, the European EHDS or the U.S. ONC framework).

The results from the AI diagnostic tests could be made clear and precise by using the FHIR (Fast Healthcare Interoperability Resources) standards which would then allow the easy transfer of data without any hitches among hospitals, laboratories, and AI analytics tools.

At the same time, the use of AI in providing feedback within EHR systems would make it possible to recommend treatments according to the patient's needs, keep track of lesions over time, and carry out predictive analytics for assessing patient risks.

6.4.6 Expanding Clinical Validation

The present case study, while confirming the therapeutic relevance of the model, nevertheless, necessitates the future investigation concerning multicenter and long-term trials.

The trials might be directed towards:

- Opening up a dialogue on the issue of model reliability for different population groups and different kinds of imaging devices.
- Trialling the communication between dermatologists and AI in writing and in the field.
- Continuous observation of the lesion for months or years through a successful collaboration between both professionals.

The commitment to extensive validation will be mandatory for regulatory approvals from such agencies as CDSCO (India), FDA (USA), or EMA (Europe), thus allowing both the commercial and clinical deployment of the model.

6.4.7 Integration of Synthetic Data and Generative AI

Specialized medical imaging still faces the challenge of data shortage. Synthetic data generation can be used for the future studies to create dermoscopic images that are not only synthetic but also realistic, using GANs or Diffusion Models, thus enriching the current datasets. If handled in an ethical manner, synthetic data can be used to balance classes, assist in the detection of rare lesions, and lower the costs of annotation. Furthermore, synthetic data generation creates opportunities for domain adaptation, allowing models trained on one population to generalize to another without the need for complete retraining.

6.4.8 Ethical AI and Policy-Driven Frameworks

AI for medicine must progress along with ethics and governance.

The future research would have to incorporate the principles of Ethics-by-Design which would ensure fairness, transparency, and accountability throughout the model lifecycle.

The main directions are:

- Charts for bias detection and mitigation will be developed for ongoing auditing.
- Explainability metrics (e.g., saliency consistency, feature attribution fidelity) will be included.
- Participation with regulatory bodies to create certification protocols for AI under NABH and CDSCO.

At the policy level, the cooperation of academic researchers, legal scholars, and health administrators will be crucial to developing frameworks that allow the coexistence of patient safety and innovation.

6.4.9 Expanding Educational and Research Impact

The study presents a remarkable groundwork for the incorporation of AI and healthcare into the academic curriculum.

Some of the possible future actions are as follows:

- Creating free learning resources or MOOCs that are modeled after this framework.
- Supporting the cross-discipline projects that involve the joint research of medical and AI students on actual datasets.
- Releasing the standard datasets and model codes for reproducibility, thus inviting worldwide research collaboration.

All these activities would be fostering the future of ethical AI professionals and speeding up the process of acceptance in both academia and healthcare institutions.

6.4.10 Cross-Domain Application Potential

The ABCNN framework, which is primarily focused on skin cancer detection, has the potential to be used in other medical imaging areas as well, such as:

- Detecting diabetic retinopathy and glaucoma (in the field of ophthalmology),
- Classifying lung nodules in chest CT scans,
- Recognizing oral lesions in dental practice, and
- Assessing wound healing in diabetic patients.

The proposed system's modular nature grants it an inherent transferability—it can be adapted to different imaging modalities with very little retraining.

Thus, a universal AI diagnostic framework, which could serve as a generalizable medical imaging platform, is created.

6.5 FINAL REMARKS

This research completion is not an end, but rather the start of a transforming journey—one that connects technology to humanity. The SegNet–ABCNN system demonstrates a change of diagnostic systems from the old, non-transparent to the new, ethical, and fair AI that can work alongside human experts.

The paper showcases that the highest level of performance in AI is of no use if not accompanied by social responsibility and inclusivity. The researchers through their painstaking experimentation reached state-of-the-art performance while keeping the conditions of privacy, fairness, and explainability intact, which are the very conditions for the sustainable healthcare innovation.

6.5.1 The Broader Impact

The combination of AI with teledermatology and public health workflows could lift healthcare access in poor areas tremendously.

Patients who used to be kept waiting for weeks to get their skin conditions checked are now getting preliminary assessments done in seconds; thus, they get the chance of early intervention and better survival rates.

The removal of geographical barriers to healthcare provision—through the use of intelligent, explainable systems—is a clear illustration of the main purpose of AI: to enhance rather than to replace human efficacy.

The model's characteristics such as being highly scalable, affordable, and interpretable add up to the cause of being a great base for the digital health revolution in India and a replicable model for other developing countries.

6.5.2 Ethical and Philosophical Reflection

Moral consideration accompanies AI, particularly in the medical field.

It is not just a combination of algorithms but also the representation of the values that have been built into them.

This study is based on the belief that AI should always be with mankind—and this means, it must be with empathy, accountability, and justice.

The project assures a future where responsible AI is accessible to all through its integration of Ethics-by-Design, transparency, and human-in-the-loop governance.

In this way, it responds to an immediate request from the academia: the need for human wisdom to direct the advancements in machine intelligence at all times.

6.5.3 Future Vision

It is predicted that automated systems such as ABCNN will become the backbone of digital healthcare networks that are integrated with one another—enabling instant communication among dermatologists, GPs, and patients in the future.

The alliance of 5G, edge computing, and federated AI are the components that can create a scenario of instantaneous worldwide health collaboration, thus eliminating the problems of distance and cost.

The rapid development of AI, IoT, and biotech is a force that makes the principles of this research—transparency, inclusivity, and interpretability—to be the ongoing guiding lights of innovation.

The aim is to reach a point where human–AI symbiosis is the reality, and the latter helps the former in the healthcare sector rather than taking over.

6.5.4 Concluding Note

The study carried out and reported in this book represents a devotion to science, compassion, and betterment of society.

It shows that AI, if it is made with good intention and care, can revamp the healthcare industry—not only as a means of maximizing productivity but also as a source of fairness and kindness.

The SegNet–ABCNN system, hence, is not only an academic contribution but also a technological proof of moral innovation—opening the door to a future where each patient no matter where he or she lives or what economic background he or she has, can get correct, prompt, and human-centered medical diagnosis.

Appendix A: Code Snippets

This appendix presents the essential code modules developed and utilized for the implementation of the proposed **SegNet–Attention-Based Convolutional Neural Network (ABCNN)** framework for skin cancer detection.

All programs were executed in *Python 3.11* with *TensorFlow 2.15* and supporting libraries, on an Ubuntu 22.04 environment equipped with an NVIDIA RTX 3060 GPU.

A.1 ENVIRONMENT SETUP

```
# Required Python libraries
tensorflow==2.15.0
keras==2.13.0
opencv-python
scikit-image
numpy
pandas
matplotlib
scikit-learn
flask
pillow
lime
tf-explain
```

A.2 PREPROCESSING UTILITIES

The preprocessing module standardizes input images through resizing, normalization, and artifact removal using the *DullRazor* technique.

```
# preprocessing.py
import cv2
import numpy as np

def resize_and_normalize(img, size=(224,224)):
    img = cv2.resize(img, size, interpolation=cv2.INTER_AREA)
    img = img.astype('float32') / 255.0
    return img

def dull_razor(img_bgr):
    """"Removes hair artifacts from dermoscopic images using morphological filtering.""""
    gray = cv2.cvtColor(img_bgr, cv2.COLOR_BGR2GRAY)
    kernel = cv2.getStructuringElement(cv2.MORPH_ELLIPSE, (9,9))
    blackhat = cv2.morphologyEx(gray, cv2.MORPH_BLACKHAT, kernel)
```

```
    _, mask = cv2.threshold(blackhat, 10, 255, cv2.THRESH_BINARY)
    mask = cv2.dilate(mask, kernel, iterations=1)
    inpaint = cv2.inpaint(img_bgr, mask, inpaintRadius=3, flags=cv2.INPAINT_TELEA)
    return inpaint

def lab_histogram_equalization(img_bgr):
    lab = cv2.cvtColor(img_bgr, cv2.COLOR_BGR2LAB)
    l, a, b = cv2.split(lab)
    l_eq = cv2.equalizeHist(l)
    lab_eq = cv2.merge((l_eq, a, b))
    return cv2.cvtColor(lab_eq, cv2.COLOR_LAB2BGR)
```

A.3 MODIFIED SEGNET ARCHITECTURE

The Modified SegNet performs lesion segmentation by isolating the region of interest (ROI) from the surrounding healthy skin tissue.

```
# segnet.py
from tensorflow.keras import layers, Model, Input

def ConvBlock(x, filters):
    x = layers.Conv2D(filters, 3, padding='same', activation='relu')(x)
    x = layers.BatchNormalization()(x)
    x = layers.Conv2D(filters, 3, padding='same', activation='relu')(x)
    x = layers.BatchNormalization()(x)
    return x

def build_modified_segnet(input_shape=(224,224,3), n_filters=[64,128,256,512]):
    inputs = Input(shape=input_shape)
    encoders = []
    x = inputs
    # Encoder path
    for f in n_filters:
        x = ConvBlock(x, f)
        encoders.append(x)
        x = layers.MaxPooling2D((2,2), padding='same')(x)
    # Bottleneck
    x = ConvBlock(x, n_filters[-1]*2)
    # Decoder path
    for idx, f in enumerate(reversed(n_filters)):
        x = layers.UpSampling2D((2,2))(x)
        x = layers.Concatenate()([x, encoders[-(idx+1)]])
        x = ConvBlock(x, f)
    outputs = layers.Conv2D(1, 1, activation='sigmoid')(x)
    return Model(inputs, outputs, name='Modified_SegNet')
```

A.4 ATTENTION-BASED CNN (ABCNN) MODEL

The **ABCNN** integrates both channel and spatial attention modules into the *Xception* backbone to enhance diagnostic interpretability.

```
# models.py
from tensorflow.keras.applications import Xception
from tensorflow.keras import layers, Model, Input
import tensorflow as tf

def channel_attention(input_feat, ratio=8):
    channel = input_feat.shape[-1]
    shared1 = layers.Dense(channel//ratio, activation='relu')
    shared2 = layers.Dense(channel)
    avg = layers.GlobalAveragePooling2D()(input_feat)
    avg = layers.Reshape((1,1,channel))(avg)
    maxp = layers.GlobalMaxPooling2D()(input_feat)
    maxp = layers.Reshape((1,1,channel))(maxp)
    avg_out = shared2(shared1(avg))
    max_out = shared2(shared1(maxp))
    cbam = layers.Add()([avg_out, max_out])
    cbam = layers.Activation('sigmoid')(cbam)
    return layers.Multiply()([input_feat, cbam])

def spatial_attention(input_feat):
    avg = tf.reduce_mean(input_feat, axis=-1, keepdims=True)
    maxp = tf.reduce_max(input_feat, axis=-1, keepdims=True)
    concat = layers.Concatenate(axis=-1)([avg, maxp])
    cbam = layers.Conv2D(1, 7, padding='same', activation='sigmoid')(concat)
    return layers.Multiply()([input_feat, cbam])

def build_abc_nn(input_shape=(224,224,3), n_classes=7):
    base = Xception(weights='imagenet', include_top=False, input_shape=input_shape)
    x = base.output
    x = channel_attention(x)
    x = spatial_attention(x)
    x = layers.GlobalAveragePooling2D()(x)
    x = layers.Dropout(0.5)(x)
    x = layers.Dense(256, activation='relu')(x)
    x = layers.BatchNormalization()(x)
    out = layers.Dense(n_classes, activation='softmax')(x)
    model = Model(inputs=base.input, outputs=out, name='ABCNN_Xception')
    return model
```

A.5 MODEL TRAINING

The following code defines image generators, augmentation strategies, and training callbacks for model convergence.

```
# train.py
import tensorflow as tf
from tensorflow.keras.preprocessing.image import ImageDataGenerator
fromtensorflow.keras.callbacksimportModelCheckpoint,EarlyStopping,ReduceLROnPlateau
```

```
def get_generators(train_dir, val_dir, target_size=(224,224), batch_size=32):
    train_aug = ImageDataGenerator(
        rescale=1./255, rotation_range=20, zoom_range=0.1,
        width_shift_range=0.1, height_shift_range=0.1,
        horizontal_flip=True, vertical_flip=True)
    val_aug = ImageDataGenerator(rescale=1./255)
    train = train_aug.flow_from_directory(train_dir, target_size=target_size,
                                          batch_size=batch_size, class_mode='categorical')
    val = val_aug.flow_from_directory(val_dir, target_size=target_size,
                                      batch_size=batch_size, class_mode='categorical')
    return train, val

def train_model(model, train, val, out_path='best_model.h5', epochs=100):
    callbacks = [
        ModelCheckpoint(out_path, monitor='val_accuracy', save_best_only=True),
        EarlyStopping(monitor='val_loss', patience=12, restore_best_weights=True),
        ReduceLROnPlateau(monitor='val_loss', factor=0.5, patience=4)
    ]
    history = model.fit(train, validation_data=val, epochs=epochs, callbacks=callbacks)
    return history
```

A.6 GRAD-CAM FOR EXPLAINABILITY

This function generates *Gradient-weighted Class Activation Maps (Grad-CAM)* to visually explain model predictions.

```
# gradcam.py
import numpy as np, tensorflow as tf, cv2
from tensorflow.keras.models import Model

def compute_gradcam(model, img_tensor, layer_name, pred_index=None):
    grad_model = Model([model.inputs], [model.get_layer(layer_name).output, model.output])
    with tf.GradientTape() as tape:
        conv_out, preds = grad_model(img_tensor)
        if pred_index is None:
            pred_index = tf.argmax(preds[0])
        class_channel = preds[:, pred_index]
    grads = tape.gradient(class_channel, conv_out)
    pooled = tf.reduce_mean(grads, axis=(0,1,2))
    conv_out = conv_out[0].numpy()
    pooled = pooled.numpy()
    for i in range(pooled.shape[0]):
        conv_out[:,:,i] *= pooled[i]
    heatmap = np.mean(conv_out, axis=-1)
    heatmap = np.maximum(heatmap,0) / np.max(heatmap)
    return cv2.resize(heatmap, (224,224))
```

A.7 FLASK-BASED WEB API FOR DEPLOYMENT

A minimal REST API using Flask allows model inference and Grad-CAM visualization through HTTP requests.

```
# app.py
from flask import Flask, request, jsonify
import tensorflow as tf, numpy as np, cv2
from preprocessing import dull_razor, resize_and_normalize
from gradcam import compute_gradcam

app = Flask(__name__)
model = tf.keras.models.load_model('abc_nn_best.h5', compile=False)
LAYER_NAME = 'block14_sepconv2'   # change to actual final conv layer

@app.route('/predict', methods=['POST'])
def predict():
    file = request.files['image']
    img = cv2.imdecode(np.frombuffer(file.read(), np.uint8), cv2.IMREAD_COLOR)
    img = dull_razor(img)
    proc = resize_and_normalize(img)
    pred = model.predict(proc[np.newaxis,...])
    cls = int(np.argmax(pred))
    conf = float(np.max(pred))
    heatmap = compute_gradcam(model, proc[np.newaxis,...], LAYER_NAME, pred_index=cls)
    return jsonify({'predicted_class': cls, 'confidence': conf})
```

A.8 UTILITY FUNCTIONS

Helper functions for evaluation metrics and saving reports.

```
# utils.py
from sklearn.metrics import classification_report, confusion_matrix
import json, numpy as np

def save_class_report(y_true, y_pred, labels, path='report.json'):
    report = classification_report(y_true, y_pred, target_names=labels, output_dict=True)
    with open(path, 'w') as f:
        json.dump(report, f, indent=2)

def save_confusion_matrix(y_true, y_pred, labels, path='confusion.npy'):
    cm = confusion_matrix(y_true, y_pred)
    np.save(path, cm)
```

A.9 NOTES

- All models were trained with **Adam optimizer (lr = 1e-4)** and **categorical cross-entropy loss**.
- Training was performed for **100 epochs** with early stopping to avoid overfitting.
- The **Grad-CAM** and **LIME** modules provided interpretability overlays aligned with dermatologist annotations.
- Quantization (FP32 → FP16) and **federated learning** setups were applied for mobile and privacy-preserving deployment (as discussed in Chapter 5).

Appendix B: Web Deployment of AI Framework

B.1 INTRODUCTION

The translation of artificial intelligence (AI) models from research environments into real-world clinical applications requires effective web deployment.

For the proposed **SegNet–Attention-Based Convolutional Neural Network (ABCNN)** architecture for automated skin cancer detection, a robust web-based deployment ensures accessibility, reproducibility, and clinical usability.

Deployment transforms a trained deep learning model into a service that can receive input (dermoscopic images), process it through the AI pipeline, and return diagnostic predictions and visual explanations (Grad-CAM, LIME).

Such deployment enables dermatologists, general practitioners, or community health workers to access AI-assisted screening remotely through web browsers or mobile devices.

B.2 OBJECTIVES OF WEB DEPLOYMENT

The deployment strategy was designed with the following objectives:

1. **Accessibility** – Provide clinicians and patients with an intuitive web interface for uploading skin lesion images and receiving results instantly.
2. **Scalability** – Ensure the system can handle multiple simultaneous requests using containerization and cloud scaling.
3. **Security and Privacy** – Enforce compliance with healthcare data protection laws such as HIPAA, GDPR, and India's Digital Personal Data Protection Act (DPDP 2023).
4. **Maintainability** – Facilitate version control, model updates, and continuous integration through Docker and cloud orchestration platforms.
5. **Explainability** – Integrate visualization layers (Grad-CAM, LIME) in the user interface to promote transparency and clinical trust.

B.3 DEPLOYMENT ARCHITECTURE

The deployment architecture for the AI-based skin cancer detection system follows a **modular, service-oriented design**, as illustrated conceptually below:

1. **Frontend Layer:**
   - Provides an intuitive graphical interface (built with HTML, React, or Flask templates).
   - Allows users to upload dermoscopic images and view Grad-CAM overlays.
   - Implements basic authentication and image anonymization before upload.
2. **Backend API Layer (Flask/FastAPI):**

- Hosts RESTful endpoints (/predict, /explain) that receive HTTP POST requests.
- Preprocesses the input image (resize, normalize, hair removal).
- Sends the processed tensor to the trained model for inference.
- Generates predictions, confidence scores, and Grad-CAM visual explanations.

3. **Model Inference Layer (TensorFlow Serving):**
   - Runs the exported SavedModel of the ABCNN on GPU-enabled cloud hardware.
   - Ensures optimized inference speed through TensorFlow Serving or ONNX Runtime.
   - Supports versioned model management for reproducibility and rollback.

4. **Storage and Logging Layer:**
   - Stores anonymized images, results, and Grad-CAM outputs in secure cloud storage (e.g., AWS S3, GCP Cloud Storage).
   - Maintains logs for each prediction (timestamp, model version, inference time, confidence).
   - Uses encryption at rest and in transit.

5. **Reverse Proxy and Load Balancer (Nginx):**
   - Routes external web requests to the Flask API through HTTPS.
   - Supports scaling across multiple containers through round-robin load balancing.
   - Integrates Let's Encrypt SSL certificates for secure access.

B.4 CONTAINERIZATION AND ORCHESTRATION

Containerization using *Docker* is central to reproducible deployment.

Each component—Flask API, TensorFlow Serving, and Nginx—is packaged into independent containers.

This approach ensures that the same environment used during development can be replicated on any server or cloud provider.

The containers can be managed collectively through **Docker Compose** for small-scale deployments or **Kubernetes (K8s)** for high availability and auto-scaling.

- *Docker Compose* allows local testing, with defined services (API, Nginx, TF-Serving) connected via internal networks.
- *Kubernetes* provides automated scaling, rolling updates, and self-healing capabilities in production.

B.5 CLOUD DEPLOYMENT OPTIONS

The model can be hosted on several cloud platforms:

Platform	Service Used	Key Benefit
Google Cloud	Cloud Run/Vertex AI	Serverless GPU scaling, native TensorFlow Serving
AWS	ECS (Fargate)/EKS	Managed containers and secure S3 integration
Microsoft Azure	App Service/AKS	Tight integration with MLOps pipelines
DigitalOcean/Heroku	App Platform	Simple deployment for research prototypes

In this research, Docker-based deployment was prioritized for its simplicity and portability, ensuring that the same container image can run locally, on a university server, or on a cloud instance with minimal modification.

B.6 WORKFLOW OF WEB DEPLOYMENT

The stepwise workflow of the web deployment process is as follows:

1. **Model Export** – The trained ABCNN model is saved in the TensorFlow SavedModel format.
2. **API Integration** – Flask application loads the model or communicates with a TensorFlow Serving instance.
3. **Containerization** – The API and model are encapsulated in a Docker image.
4. **Reverse Proxy Setup** – Nginx routes requests and enforces HTTPS security.
5. **Testing and Benchmarking** – The system is tested using dermoscopic images for latency, accuracy, and reliability.
6. **Deployment to Cloud** – The container is uploaded to a cloud registry and deployed on a hosting platform.
7. **Monitoring and Maintenance** – Logs, errors, and metrics are continuously monitored for system health and model drift.

B.7 SECURITY AND COMPLIANCE

Healthcare AI deployment demands strict adherence to privacy, data protection, and ethical use.

The deployed web service therefore incorporates multiple safeguards:

- **Data Encryption:** All communication uses HTTPS with TLS 1.3.
- **Anonymization:** Metadata such as patient names or IDs are removed before upload.
- **Access Control:** User authentication is implemented through secure tokens.
- **Audit Logging:** Every prediction is logged with a model version identifier.
- **Regulatory Compliance:** The system complies with HIPAA, GDPR, and DPDP Act (India, 2023).
- **Federated Learning Readiness:** For future updates, the architecture supports local model training at distributed sites without transferring raw patient data.

B.8 SCALABILITY AND MAINTENANCE

The AI inference layer can be scaled horizontally by increasing the number of containers or instances based on incoming requests.

A **load balancer** distributes traffic among servers, ensuring responsiveness during peak load.

Continuous integration and deployment (CI/CD) pipelines can automate model updates when new data or retrained models become available.

Model Versioning:

- Version control ensures that every model deployed has a unique ID.
- Old models can be rolled back instantly if performance issues arise.

Performance Monitoring:

- Logging frameworks such as *Prometheus* or *Grafana* can track latency and throughput.
- Regular A/B testing allows benchmarking of new versions against deployed baselines.

B.9 ETHICAL CONSIDERATIONS

AI deployment in healthcare carries significant ethical responsibility.

Transparency, fairness, and accountability are embedded in the design of this deployment framework.

By integrating explainable AI visualizations (Grad-CAM and LIME) directly into the web interface, clinicians are empowered to verify model logic rather than blindly trust predictions.

This transparency promotes **trustworthy AI**, aligning with the **WHO (2021)** and **EU AI Act (2024)** guidelines for ethical AI in medicine.

B.10 CONCLUSION

The deployment of the proposed **SegNet–ABCNN** model as a secure, scalable, and explainable web service marks the crucial step from research innovation to clinical applicability.

Through a modular, containerized architecture, the system ensures robustness, reproducibility, and accessibility even in resource-limited healthcare settings.

The web deployment not only provides **real-time diagnostic support** but also sets a foundation for **nationwide teledermatology integration** under India's *Ayushman Bharat Digital Health Mission (ABDM).*

With continued refinements in privacy-preserving learning and cloud optimization, the system has the potential to evolve into a national-level screening platform for early skin cancer detection.

Bibliography

S. Agale, V. Bhatia, G. DCosta, and B. Bharambe, "Childhood actinic keratosis in an albino transforming into squamous cell carcinoma," *Indian Dermatology Online Journal*, vol. 3, no. 3, p. 199, 2012.

M. Agarwal, K. S. Gill, P. Aggarwal, R. S. Rawat, and G. Sunil, "Urban sound classification using vgg19 convolutional neural network (cnn) model and its visualisation," in *2024 4th International Conference on Innovative Practices in Technology and Management (ICIPTM)*. IEEE, 2024, pp. 1–5.

P. Agrahari, A. Agrawal, and N. Subhashini, "Skin cancer detection using deep learning," in *Futuristic Communication and Network Technologies, VICFCNT*. Singapore: Springer, 2022.

A. F. Ahamed, Y. Sukhi, K. S. Lasya, P. Karishma, and M. Priyankha, "Unity power factor operation for non linear load applications using interleaved Manitoba rectifier," in *2022 International Interdisciplinary Humanitarian Conference for Sustainability (IIHC)*. IEEE, Nov. 2022.

V. Ahlgrimm-Siess, R. G. B. Langley, and R. Hofmann-Wellenhof, "Solar lentigo, seborrheic keratosis and lichen planus-like keratosis," in *Reflectance Confocal Microscopy for Skin Diseases*. Springer Berlin Heidelberg, 2011, pp. 259–270.

S. Albahli, M. Masud, H. Alhumyani, and T. Alshammari, "A multimodal approach for early detection of skin cancer using deep learning," *Neural Computing and Applications*, vol. 34, pp. 16 793–16 802, 2022.

A. M. H. Alhussainy, "A new pooling layer based on wavelet transform for convolutional neural network," *Journal of Advanced Research in Dynamical and Control Systems*, vol. 24, no. 4, pp. 76–85, Mar. 2020.

V. R. Allugunti, "A machine learning model for skin disease classification using convolutional neural network," *International Journal of Computer Programming and Database Management*, vol. 2, pp. 141–147, 2022.

U. B. Ansari and T. Sarode, "Skin cancer detection using image processing," *International Research Journal of Engineering and Technology (IRJET)*, vol. 4, no. 4, pp. 2875–2881, 2017.

A. Bhattacharya, A. Young, S. Stalling, D. Hadley, A. Wong, and M. Wei, "Precision diagnosis of melanoma and other skin lesions from digital images," *AMIA Summits on Translational Science Proceedings*, vol. 2017, no. Suppl 2, pp. 220–226, 2017.

M. Brggen and G. Stingl, "Subcutaneous white adipose tissue: The deepest layer of the cutaneous immune barrier," *Journal Der Deutschen Dermatologischen Gesellschaft (JDDG)*, vol. 18, no. 11, pp. 1225–1227, 2020.

T. J. Brinker et al., "Skin cancer classification using convolutional neural networks: Systematic review," *Journal of Medical Internet Research*, vol. 20, no. 10, p. e11936, 2018.

T. J. Brinker, A. Hekler, A. H. Enk, C. Berking, S. Haferkamp, A. Hauschild, M.Weichenthal, J. Klode, D. Schadendorf, T. Holland-Letz, and J. S. Utikal, "Deep neural networks are superior to dermatologists in melanoma image classification," in *European Academy of Dermatology and Venereology (EADV)*, 2019.

M. Camara, V. L. Rocha De Sousa, P. M. Pinheiro, P. D. T. Neto, J. Costa, and R. Jales, "Multiple dermatofibromas: Dermoscopic patterns," *Indian Journal of Dermatology*, vol. 58, no. 3, p. 243, 2013.

S. Chatterjee, B. Mukhopadhyay, A. Shukla, O. Speck, A. Das, C. Sarasaen, A. Nrnberger, C. Mandal, M. Vipinraj, and R. Nagaraja Rao, "Torchesegeta: Framework for interpretability and explainability of image-based deep learning models," *Applied Sciences*, vol. 12, no. 4, p. 1834, 2022.

S. S. Chaturvedi, K. Gupta, and P. S. Prasad, "Skin lesion analyser: An efficient seven way multiclass skin cancer classification using mobilenet," in *Advanced Machine Learning Technologies and Applications, ser. Advances in Intelligent Systems and Computing*. Springer, 2020, vol. 1141, pp. 86–97.

S. S. Chaturvedi, J. V. Tembhurne, and T. Diwan, "A multiclass skin cancer classification using deep convolutional neural networks," *Multimedia Tools and Applications*, vol. 79, no. 39-40, pp. 28 477–28 498, 2020.

J. Y. Chen, K. Fernandez, R. P. Fadadu, R. Reddy, M.-O. Kim, J. Tan, and M. L. Wei, "Skin cancer diagnosis by lesion, physician, and examination type," *JAMA Dermatology*, vol. 161, no. 2, p. 135, 2024.

M. Chen, W. Chen, W. Chen, L. Cai, and G. Chai, "Skin cancer classification with deep convolutional neural networks," *Journal of Medical Imaging and Health Informatics*, vol. 10, no. 7, pp. 1707–1713, 2020.

N. C. Codella, Q. B. Nguyen, S. Pankanti, D. Gutman, B. Helba, A. Halpern, and J. R. Smith, "Deep learning ensembles for melanoma recognition in dermoscopy images," *IBM Journal of Research and Development*, vol. 61, no. 4/5, pp. 5:1–5:15, 2017.

A. Dascalu and E. O. David, "Skin cancer detection by deep learning and sound analysis algorithms: a prospective clinical study of an elementary dermoscope," *eBioMedicine*, vol. 43, pp. 107–113, 2019.

O. Demirel and M. T. Akhtar, "Dual-input type convolutional neural networks employing color normalized and nuclei segmented data for histopathology image classification," in *2023 IEEE Statistical Signal Processing Workshop (SSP)*. IEEE, Jul. 2023.

U.-O. Dorj, K.-K. Lee, J.-Y. Choi, and M. Lee, "The skin cancer classification using deep convolutional neural network," *Multimedia Tools and Applications*, vol. 77, no. 8, pp. 9909–9924, 2018.

T. Emara, H. M. Afify, F. H. Ismail, and A. E. Hassanien, "A modified inceptionv4 for imbalanced skin cancer classification dataset," in *2019 14th International Conference on Computer Engineering and Systems (ICCES)*. IEEE, 2019, pp. 28–33.

N. S. A. Eneze and A. L. Kolifi, "A method of skin disease detection using image processing and machine learning," *Procedia Computer Science*, vol. 163, pp. 85–92, 2019.

A. Esteva, B. Kuprel, R. A. Novoa, J. Ko, S. M. Swetter, H. M. Blau, and S. Thrun, "Dermatologist-level classification of skin cancer with deep neural networks," *Nature*, vol. 542, pp. 115–118, 2017.

N. Gessert, M. Nielsen, M. Shaikh, R. Werner, and A. Schlaefer, "Skin lesion classification using ensembles of multi-resolution efficient nets with meta data," *Methods*, vol. 179, pp. 46–58, 2020.

M. Goyal, A. Oakley, A. Bansal, D. Dancey, and M. H. Yap, "Skin lesion segmentation in dermoscopic images with ensemble deep learning methods," *IEEE Access*, vol. 8, pp. 4171–4181, 2020.

B. Harangi, "Skin lesion classification with ensembles of deep convolutional neural networks," *Journal of Biomedical Informatics*, vol. 86, pp. 25–32, 2018.

A. Hekler, J. S. Utikal, A. H. Enk et al., "Superior skin cancer classification by the combination of human and artificial intelligence," *European Journal of Cancer*, vol. 120, pp. 114–121, 2019.

L. Hoang, S. H. Lee, E. J. Lee, and K. R. Kwon, "Multiclass skin lesion classification using a novel lightweight deep learning framework for smart healthcare," *Applied Sciences*, vol. 12, no. 5, p. 2677, 2022.

K. M. Hosny, M. A. Kassem, and M. M. Foaud, "Skin cancer classification using deep learning and transfer learning," in *2018 9th Cairo International Biomedical Engineering Conference (CIBEC)*. IEEE, 2018, pp. 90–93.

W. Hu, R. Ni, L. Fang, G. Pan, and H. Zhang, "Changing trends in the disease burden of non-melanoma skin cancer globally from 1990 to 2019 and its predicted level in 25 years," *BMC Cancer*, vol. 22, no. 1, 2022. [Online]. Available: https://doi.org/10.1186/s12885-022-09940-3

Y. S. Ingle and N. F. Shaikh, "Review on skin cancer detection using ai," *International Journal of Health Sciences*, vol. 6, no. S2, 2022.

Y. S. Ingle and N. F. Shaikh, "Skin cancer recognition using cnn, vgg16 and vgg19," in *ICT for Intelligent Systems, ICTIS*. Singapore: Springer, 2023.

M. T. Islam, M. A. Aowal, A. T. Minhaz, and K. Ashraf, "Skin cancer detection using deep learning approach," *International Journal of Advanced Computer Science and Applications*, vol. 8, no. 10, pp. 347–353, 2017.

H. Iyatomi, H. Oka, M. E. Celebi, M. Hashimoto, M. Tanaka, M. Hagiwara, and K. Ogawa, "An improved internet-based melanoma screening system with dermatologist-like tumor area extraction algorithm," *Computerized Medical Imaging and Graphics*, vol. 32, no. 7, pp. 566–579, 2008.

S. Jinnai, N. Yamazaki, Y. Hirano, Y. Sugawara, Y. Ohe, and R. Hamamoto, "The development of a skin cancer classification system for pigmented skin lesions using deep learning," *Biomolecules*, vol. 10, no. 8, p. 1123, 2020.

M. A. Khan, T. Akram, M. Sharif, S. Kadry, and V. Rajinikanth, "A framework of deep learning for diagnosis of skin cancer using transfer learning," *Journal of Ambient Intelligence and Humanized Computing*, vol. 12, pp. 7957–7978, 2021.

M. A. Khan, N. Hussain, A. Majid, M. Sharif, M. Raza, T. Saba, and A. Rehman, "Classification of dermoscopy images for early diagnosis of skin cancer using hybrid features," *Microscopy Research and Technique*, vol. 84, no. 5, pp. 1079–1090, 2021.

S. Kortam, I. Metanes, J. Krausz, A. Kramer, D. Weihs, Y. Har-Shai, D. Ad-El, and Y. Merkher, "Rapid, quantitative prediction of tumor invasiveness in non-melanoma skin cancers using mechanobiology-based assay," *Biomechanics and Modeling in Mechanobiology*, vol. 20, no. 5, pp. 1767–1774, 2021.

K. Liu, G. Kang, N. Zhang, and B. Hou, "Breast cancer classification based on fully-connected layer first convolutional neural networks," *IEEE Access*, vol. 6, pp. 23 722–23 732, 2018.

J. A. V. Lpez, D. A. M. D. ngel, J. A. E. Gonzlez, A. Padilla, and M. D. L. M. Ferretiz, "Case report: Mustard flap perform for reconstruction of the cheek in a patient with basal cell carcinoma in a second level of care," *International Journal of Medical Science and Clinical Research Studies*, vol. 4, no. 11, 2024.

A. Mahbod, G. Schaefer, C. Wang, R. Ecker, I. Ellinger, A. Pitiot, and Y. Yuan, "Transfer learning using a multi-scale and multi-network ensemble for skin lesion classification," *Computer Methods and Programs in Biomedicine*, vol. 193, p. 105475, 2020.

K. Mahbubani, "The world health organization (who)," *Global Public Health*, vol. 7, no. 3, pp. 312–314, 2012.

N. Marini, M. Atzori, S. Otalora, S. Marchand-Maillet, and H. Muller, "H&Eadversarial network: a convolutional neural network to learn stain-invariant features through hematoxylin & eosin regression," in *2021 IEEE/CVF International Conference on Computer Vision Workshops (ICCVW)*. IEEE, Oct. 2021.

A. Menegola, M. Fornaciali, R. Pires, S. Avila, and E. Valle, "Knowledge transfer for melanoma screening with deep learning," in *2017 IEEE 14th International Symposium on Biomedical Imaging (ISBI)*. IEEE, 2017, pp. 297–300.

R. M. Merrill, "Risk-adjusted melanoma skin cancer incidence rates in whites (united states)," *Melanoma Research*, vol. 21, no. 6, pp. 535–540, 2011.

I. D. Mienye, G. Obaido, M. Jordan, T. G. Swart, and P. Ilono, "Deep convolutional neural networks in medical image analysis: A review," *Information*, vol. 16, no. 3, p. 195, 2025.

A. Mobiny, A. Singh, and H. Van Nguyen, "Risk-aware machine learning classifier for skin lesion diagnosis," *Journal of Clinical Medicine*, vol. 8, no. 8, p. 1241, 2019.

S. Mohapatra, N. V. S. Abhishek, D. Bardhan, A. A. Ghosh, and S. Mohanty, "Skin cancer classification using convolution neural networks," in *Advances in Distributed Computing and Machine Learning, ser. Lecture Notes in Networks and Systems*. Springer, 2021, vol. 127 .

H. Nahata and S. P. Singh, "Deep learning solutions for skin cancer detection and diagnosis," in *Machine Learning with Health Care Perspective*. Cham: Springer, 2020, p. 13.

N. V. A. O. Nancy, P. Arya, and M. S. Arya, "Comparative study and analysis on skin cancer detection using machine learning and deep learning algorithms," *Multimedia Tools and Applications*, vol. 82, pp. 45 913–45 957, 2023.

E. Nasr-Esfahani, S. Samavi, N. Karimi, S. M. Soroushmehr, M. H. Jafari, K. R. Ward, and K. Najarian, "Melanoma detection by analysis of clinical images using convolutional neural network," in *Conference Proceedings of the IEEE Engineering in Medicine and Biology Society*, pp. 1373–1376, 2016.

M. Nauta, R. Walsh, A. Dubowski, and C. Seifert, "Uncovering and correcting shortcut learning in machine learning models for skin cancer diagnosis," *Diagnostics*, vol. 12, no. 1, p. 40, 2022.

I. A. Ozkan and M. Koklu, "Skin lesion classification using machine learning algorithms," *International Journal of Intelligent Systems and Applications in Engineering*, vol. 5, pp. 285–289, 2017.

P. Pasquali and M. J. Gutirrez, "Cryosurgery for vascular lesions," in *CryosurgeryA Practical Manual*. Springer Berlin Heidelberg, 2014, pp. 143–156.

A. Patil, Y. S. Ingle, N. F. Shaikh, P. Mahalle, and J. Barot, "Skin cancer image augmentation techniques using ai: A survey of the state-of-the-art," in *ICT Infrastructure and Computing, ICT4SD*. Singapore: Springer, 2023.

K.-C. Peng and T. Chen, "Cross-layer features in convolutional neural networks for generic classification tasks," in *2015 IEEE International Conference on Image Processing (ICIP)*. IEEE, Sep. 2015.

P. M. Pereira, R. Fonseca-Pinto, R. P. Paiva, P. Assuncao, A. Monteiro, I. N. Figueiredo, and H. P. Oliveira, "Skin lesion classification enhancement using borderline featuresthe dermatologist criteria," *Sensors*, vol. 20, no. 5, p. 1431, 2020.

T. C. Pham, G. S. Tran, T. P. Nghiem, A. Doucet, C. M. Luong, and V.-D. Hoang, "A comparative study for classification of skin cancer," in *2019 International Conference on System Science and Engineering (ICSSE)*. IEEE, 2019, pp. 267–272.

S. Pop, O. Urtatiz, and C. Van Raamsdonk, "Isolation of tdtomato expressing inter-follicular epidermal melanocytes or keratinocytes from mouse tail skin," *Bio-Protocol*, vol. 12, no. 8, 2022.

M. Rashid, S. Sulaiman, R. Karim, and A. Salman, "Improved skin lesion segmentation using the saliency detection approach," *Symmetry*, vol. 11, no. 2, p. 242, 2019.

S. Serte and H. Demirel, "Gabor wavelet-based deep learning for skin lesion classification," *Computers in Biology and Medicine*, vol. 103, pp. 264–271, 2018.

J. Shaikh, R. Khan, Y. S. Ingle, and N. F. Shaikh, "Improved skin cancer detection using cnn," *International Journal of Health Sciences*, vol. 6, no. S2, 2022.

J. Shaikh, R. Khan, Y. Ingle, and N. F. Shaikh, "Skin cancer detection: A review using ai techniques," *International Journal of Health Sciences*, vol. 6, no. S2, 2022.

G. Stinco, E. Errichetti, and A. Lallas, "Melanocytic nevi," in *Dermatoscopy and Skin Cancer*. CRC Press, 2021, pp. 124–130.

J. V. Tembhurne, N. Hebbar, and H. Y. Patil, "Skin cancer detection using ensemble of machine learning and deep learning techniques," *Multimedia Tools and Applications*, vol. 82, pp. 27 501–27 524, 2023.

K. Thurnhofer-Hemsi, E. Lpez-Rubio, E. Domnguez, and D. Elizondo, "Skin lesion classification by ensembles of deep convolutional networks and regularly spaced shifting," *IEEE Access*, vol. 9, pp. 112 193–112 205, 2021.

K. Uchida, M. Tanaka, and M. Okutomi, "Coupled convolution layer for convolutional neural network," in *2016 23rd International Conference on Pattern Recognition (ICPR)*. IEEE, Dec. 2016.

V. Verma, A. Khan, and S. Tiwari, "Traffic signs classification using convolutional neural network (CNN)," in *Proceedings of the 3rd International Conference on Advanced Computing and Software Engineering*. SCITEPRESS – Science and Technology Publications, 2021.

M. M. Vijayalakshmi, "Melanoma skin cancer detection using image processing and machine learning," *International Journal of Trend in Scientific Research and Development (IJTSRD)*, vol. 3, no. 4, pp. 780–784, 2019.

E. Yilmaz and E. Ekinci, "Skin lesion classification using modified deep learning techniques," *Medical Biological Engineering Computing*, vol. 59, pp. 2483–2495, 2021.

L. Yu, H. Chen, Q. Dou, J. Qin, and P.-A. Heng, "Automated melanoma recognition in dermoscopy images via very deep residual networks," *IEEE Transactions on Medical Imaging*, vol. 36, no. 4, pp. 994–1004, 2017.

Index

For Product Safety Concerns and Information please contact our
EU representative GPSR@taylorandfrancis.com Taylor & Francis
Verlag GmbH, Kaufingerstraße 24, 80331 München, Germany